365 Days Social Posts for Dentistry

RACHEL MELE

DEDICATION

Proceeds from this book are being donated to Oral Cancer Cause, an organization dedicated to improving the quality of life for oral cancer patients through financial support so they may face the world with peace and dignity during and after medical treatment.

ACKNOWLEDGMENTS

Mom, you are the most inspiring person in my life. You have been the best role model anyone could ask for. Thank you for introducing me to this profession. Thank you for empowering me to know I make good decisions. And, of course, thank you for the hours you dedicated to helping me make this book a reality.

Dad, this book wouldn't be possible had I not inherited your incredible work-ethic! You are my superhero.

Jeff. I love you. I remember the day, shortly after we started dating, I told you I had purchased the domain name www.rachelmele.com. I always knew you were the one for me. You are the most brilliant person I have ever met. You are an incredible husband and the most amazing father to our children. Thank you for always believing in me.

Fabiana, my research assistant. Thank you. Without you, this book would not have become a reality.

Sesameeps, thank you for an amazing ten years, and for giving me a platform to educate and help grow thousands of dental practices.

Diana Friedman for recognizing my talents and pushing me to be the best person I can be.

Linda Miles, thank you for educating our profession about the importance of oral cancer screenings through your foundation, Oral Cancer Cause. I pray the proceeds from this book makes the lives of those suffering from oral cancer a little bit easier.

Aunt Rachel. You are my spiritual guidance and inspiration.

Thank you to everyone in the dental profession who has supported me along the way. There are too many to name, but you know who you are.

INTRODUCTION

In 2006, I started collecting dental-themed social media posts from across the world. I relentlessly followed and liked every dentist, dental specialist, dental magazine and dental manufacturer I could find. My social feeds were (and still are) filled with dental posts of every kind. Some were funny, like a dentist signing a popular tune with comical dental lyrics (love that). Others educated me on the importance of oral cancer screening, or the heart/mouth connection. One time a dentist's social posts about his technology led me to schedule an appointment with his practice for my son. Now our entire family goes to that dentist. Occasionally a post was so engaging, I would comment on or share what I saw. Of course, mixed in with those head-of-the-class social posts, were a lot of non-engaging, make me snore, "I may have to unlike this practice" posts. But when I saw one I found particularly interesting, funny, or engaging, I put it in a folder I called "365." Over the years, I would write articles about the best dental social posts I had read. I would share them with my dental clients and during lectures to encourage practices to "beef up" their social engagement. I always had it on my bucket list to turn the best of the best into a book that could be used by any dental practice or specialty. "365 Days of Social Posts for Dentistry" is my collection from the last decade.

My hope is your dental marketing team will read this book and use it as a template to guide you to create your own funny, informative, educational and, most importantly, engaging social media posts. The template is set up with three parts. The first section, at the top of each page, includes an idea. You could certainly copy and paste the text and use it as is, but I highly recommend making it your own. The second section provides a description with suggestions on how to personalize those posts. These are meant to spark your creative side. Use the description to come up with your own unique videos, photographs, imagery, blogs and stories that connect your patients and prospective patients to your practice. The third section is a link to a related example.

As you create your own unique posts, feel free to share them with me or post them yourself using the hashtag #365SocialDentistry Join me on my mission to inspire friends, family, community and the greater population to educate one another by innovating solutions that make it easier to stay engaged and connected. Innovations that improve personal health, happiness, and fulfillment globally. Dentists are the only oral physicians of the mouth. By educating, through social media and other forms of communication and collaboration every day, we all can improve the health and happiness of patients around the world.

Happy New Year

SAY THIS

Happy New Year! New goals, new memories to be made and new insurance benefits to be used! Schedule your routine checkup & cleaning for healthier gums & teeth!

,,

DESCRIPTION

Say Happy New Year to your patients! Get creative with a picture of your team or a New Year graphic.

LINK: **WWW.RACHELMELE.COM/1-1**

New Year Resolutions

SAY THIS

Here are some dental New Year's resolutions we heard from our patients. 1. Brush two times, two minutes per day. 2. Floss everyday. 3. Visit my dentist at least twice a year.

What's your dental resolution?

99

DESCRIPTION

Write your own dental blog and post your own New Year's resolution ideas or link to articles like the one below.

LINK: **WWW.RACHELMELE.COM/1-2**

Patient Feature

SAY THIS

Look who came to visit us for a cleaning.
Schedule your appointment today!

99

DESCRIPTION

Feature a picture of one of your patients and include a funny caption to get a couple giggles from your followers! See the example below.

LINK: **WWW.RACHELMELE.COM/1-3**

National Trivia Day

SAY THIS

It's National Trivia Day. Teeth have many layers and components including

_____.

A) Nerves B) Muscles C) Veins D) Joints

99

DESCRIPTION

It's National Trivia Day! Share a dental trivia question with your followers to get the conversation started. Post the answer to your Trivia Question at the end of the day.

LINK: **WWW.RACHELMELE.COM/1-4**

Team Appreciation

SAY THIS

Today, we are featuring our Team Member of the Month, [Team Member Name], our receptionist. We love how [Team Member Name] greets every patient with a smile. Thanks [Team Member Name] for taking such great care of our patients.

,,

DESCRIPTION

It's important to highlight your staff and make them feel appreciated. By showing off an employee each month, your followers will get to know the team better.

LINK: **WWW.RACHELMELE.COM/1-5**

National Technology Day

SAY THIS

It's National Technology Day. In honor of this day, we want to share our coolest dental technology, our Solea Laser. Learn more about it here.

,,

DESCRIPTION

Show off your latest gadget. Or, display an article of an innovative dental technology product you are interested in and ask your followers who would like to use it!

LINK: **WWW.RACHELMELE.COM/1-6**

Question

SAY THIS

According to the Academy of General Dentistry, the average person only brushes for 45 to 70 seconds a day. How much time do you take to brush your teeth each day?

"

DESCRIPTION

Ask your followers a question regarding their dental habits to open the door to conversation. Make sure you respond to their answers!

LINK: WWW.RACHELMELE.COM/1-7

Quote

SAY THIS

"A laugh is a smile that bursts."

~Mary H. Waldrip

99

DESCRIPTION

A dental quote that followers can relate to can put a smile on their face! Choose your quotes wisely!

LINK: **WWW.RACHELMELE.COM/1-8**

Dental Joke

Our practice joke of the day:

Q: What did the tooth say to the departing dentist?

Comment what you think the answer might be!

"

DESCRIPTION

A: Fill me in when you get back.
Write the answer in a comment
after you have several answers.

LINK: WWW.RACHELMELE.COM/1-9

Question

SAY THIS

Have you had a good experience at [Practice Name]? We'd love for you to share an experience or memory!

"

DESCRIPTION

Encourage followers to comment on your posts by asking them questions. Respond to those who comment and make them feel like their opinion matters!

LINK: **WWW.RACHELMELE.COM/1-10**

Blog About Food

SAY THIS

Want healthier gums? Eat more of these foods: [Include Article Link]

"

DESCRIPTION

Write a blog post on healthy foods to eat to benefit your gums!

LINK: **WWW.RACHELMELE.COM/1-11**

Dental Fun

SAY THIS

We are taking a vote. Ask your kids if we should
add these slinkies to our treasure chest?

,,

DESCRIPTION

Provide an image of an item you are
considering adding to your toy box.

LINK: WWW.RACHELMELE.COM/1-12

SnapChat

SAY THIS

*Today [Practice Doctor Name] and
[Patient Name] said hello to face swap!
SAY CHEESE!*

"

DESCRIPTION

Download snapchat and have fun with
the face swap filter.

LINK: WWW.RACHELMELE.COM/1-13

Dental Games

SAY THIS

Kids will spend time playing games, make sure they are good ones... Check out "Bad Teeth Makeover."

,,

DESCRIPTION

Post a link to your favorite dental related online game.

LINK: **WWW.RACHELMELE.COM/1-14**

MLK DAY

SAY THIS

Martin Luther King, Jr. once said, "life's most persistent and urgent question is, what are you doing for others?" At [Practice Name] we help our patients feel good and love their smile! Happy Martin Luther King, Jr. Day!

"

DESCRIPTION

It's Martin Luther King Jr. Day of Service. Today Americans across the country come together to serve their neighbors and communities. Remind followers about this special day with a quote from MLK and a personalized touch of your practice.

LINK: **WWW.RACHELMELE.COM/1-15**

Customer Review

SAY THIS

Check out this video of [Patient Name] saying great things about our practice! We love our patients!

,,

DESCRIPTION

Record a quick video of one of your patients leaving a great video review about the practice! Don't forget to tag them and get written permission to do so.

LINK: WWW.RACHELMELE.COM/1-16

No Nail Biting

SAY THIS

*Say **NO** to nail biting, or you will say **YES** to this: grinding and clenching your teeth, chipping your teeth, cuts to your gums, and gingivitis.*

,,

DESCRIPTION

Write your own dental blog post on the negatives of nail biting habits.

LINK: **WWW.RACHELMELE.COM/1-17**

Dental Tips

SAY THIS

If you knock out a tooth, here are some steps that may help ensure we can save it. 1) don't touch the root of the tooth, 2) rinse it off with milk if dirty, 3) keep it moist by dropping it into a glass of milk, 4) get to our office quickly.

"

DESCRIPTION

Provide tips and tricks that can come in handy to followers. Share the wealth of dental knowledge!

LINK: **WWW.RACHELMELE.COM/1-18**

Get to Know Your Customers Day

SAY THIS

[Insert picture of patient] Happy National Get to Know Your Customers Day! This is [Patient name]. [He/She] enjoys [hobby] in [his/her] free time. [He/She] visits [Practice Name] because [reason why patient visits your practice].

"

DESCRIPTION

Take a picture of one of your happiest patients! Ask them a couple questions and ask them if they would like to be featured.

LINK: **WWW.RACHELMELE.COM/1-19**

Quote

SAY THIS

"Beauty is power; a smile is its sword."

~John Ray

DESCRIPTION

Do a Google search for "dental quotes" to find more great examples to post throughout the year.

Patient Feature

SAY THIS

Check out our patient [Patient's Name].
[He/She] recently got Veneers®/or

_____.

Look what it did for [his/ her] smile!

"

DESCRIPTION

It's great to let your followers know the perks of the services you provide! Feature a picture of a patient's smile that benefits from a product or service your practice performed. Use full face photos, if possible.

LINK: **WWW.RACHELMELE.COM/1-21**

Team Appreciation

SAY THIS

Hello from [Team Member's Name] at the front desk. [Team Member's Name] will greet you when you come into our practice. Call to make your appointment with [Team member's Name] today or just to say hello!

DESCRIPTION

Capture a photo of your front desk team member! A perfect way to remind patients or future patients your practice is a friendly and welcoming environment.

LINK: **WWW.RACHELMELE.COM/1-22**

Video

SAY THIS

Check out this singing dentist rocking to his version of "Wanna Be Startin Something" by Michael Jackson.

,,

DESCRIPTION

Add or create your own
video to link to this post.

LINK: **WWW.RACHELMELE.COM/1-23**

Contest

SAY THIS

Who do you know that wears the best socks? Tag them here to enter them to win a pair of teeth socks from [Practice Name].

,,

DESCRIPTION

Winners could be patients or not yet patients. Include a link to these awesome teeth socks.

LINK: WWW.RACHELMELE.COM/1- 24

Practice Promotion

SAY THIS

New Patient Promotion! Don't hate going to the dentist ever again! Low-cost, no obligation promotion starts today and lasts through the end of the month!

"

DESCRIPTION

Use word or pages to make a graphic of a new patient promotion to go along with your post. See example below. Limit sales posts to a few a quarter.

LINK: **WWW.RACHELMELE.COM/1-25**

Spouse Day Fun

SAY THIS

Happy Spouse's Day to all our patients' significant others! Has your spouse been to our office in the last six months? If not, give us a call to schedule an appointment, we want them to have a great smile for you. [Practice Phone #]

,,

DESCRIPTION

Post a picture dedicated to the spouses in the practice. This is also a funny reminder directed to all the "wifeys" looking out for their "hubbys". Consider posting a link to schedule online.

LINK: **WWW.RACHELMELE.COM/1-26**

Tooth Organizer

SAY THIS

Who said you had to throw out your baby teeth? Check out this Kids Tooth Box Organizer that could make a great gift from the tooth fairy!

,,

DESCRIPTION

Expose followers to innovative and fun products they could use, such as this Kids Tooth Box Organizer!

LINK: WWW.RACHELMELE.COM/1-27

National Fun at Work Day

SAY THIS

Today is National Fun at Work Day!
Working with such a great team makes everyday
fun, don't you agree?

"

DESCRIPTION

Take photos throughout the day of fun
and silly moments team members have.

LINK: **WWW.RACHELMELE.COM/1-28**

Doctor Appreciation

SAY THIS

Meet our Doctors: [Doctor(s) Name]

They make our practice great.

99

DESCRIPTION

Introduce your doctors to your social media followers! You can do this by taking a picture of them individually or a group picture. Make sure your followers know you appreciate the doctors(s)' outstanding skills.

LINK: WWW.RACHELMELE.COM/1-29

Quote

SAY THIS

This is [Doctor's Name's] favorite quote. "It takes 17 muscles to smile and 43 to frown." ~Author Unknown

"

DESCRIPTION

Ask the doctors in your practice what their favorite dental quote is and post it here or take a video of them saying why it's special.

LINK: WWW.RACHELMELE.COM/1-30

Invisalign®
Promotion

SAY THIS

We find that Invisalign® aligners are most effective when worn 20 to 22 hours per day and removed only for eating, brushing and flossing. Are you on track?

,,

DESCRIPTION

It's great to let your followers know the perks of the services you provide! Talk these products up and let them know why they should come to your practice to have this service done.

LINK: **WWW.RACHELMELE.COM/1-31**

Children's Health Month

SAY THIS

Developing good habits early on, along with regular dental visits, will help children get a good start on a lifetime of healthy gums and teeth. Has your child visited us in the past six months? If not, it's time to give us a call and schedule an appointment. [Practice Phone #].

"

DESCRIPTION

Remind patients to schedule their regular check-ups. Consider including a link to a blog post about good dental habits.

LINK: WWW.RACHELMELE.COM/2-1

Groundhog Day

SAY THIS

Happy Groundhog day! Fun dental fact: Groundhogs have four incisors, shaped like chisels, two upper and two lower. The upper two continue to grow at the rate of 1/16 of an inch every week!

,,

DESCRIPTION

It's Groundhog Day. Remind your patients of this by including a dental fact about groundhogs like the example below.

LINK: WWW.RACHELMELE.COM/ 2-2

Tooth Brushes

SAY THIS

[Practice Name] recommends the following children's tooth brushes and tooth paste: [Fill-in the blank]. Click on the link below to read why!

,,

DESCRIPTION

Write your own dental blog post on the best toothbrushes for kids or link to your article!

LINK: **WWW.RACHELMELE.COM/2-3**

Early Valentine's Day Promotion

SAY THIS

Valentine's Day is close! Surprise your significant other with a teeth whitening from our practice! Give us a call, and we'll send you a gift certificate.

99

DESCRIPTION

Give couples a fresh idea for Valentine's Day! Advertise free time slots for couples to come in and get their teeth whitened, or a special couple deal!

LINK: **WWW.RACHELMELE.COM/ 2-4**

Dental Games

SAY THIS

Educate your kids about good oral hygiene. Try Colgate® Kids tooth games and activities.

,,

DESCRIPTION

Parents are always looking for online resources to educate their kids! This is a great tool to encourage positive dental health.

LINK: **WWW.RACHELMELE.COM/2-5**

American Heart Month

SAY THIS

February is American Heart Month. It's true—a healthy mouth promotes a healthy heart!

,,

DESCRIPTION

Write your own dental blog post on how heart disease links to gum disease. For ideas, check out this post from this dental practice!

LINK: **WWW.RACHELMELE.COM/2-6**

Picture Sharing

SAY THIS

Let's share the laughter! Post your (or your kid's) post-dentist pictures. The funnier, the better! Ready, set, post! Be sure to tag us.

99

DESCRIPTION

Highlight funny pictures and comments on all posts. Be sure to mention this request to patients while they are in the office, too.

LINK: **WWW.RACHELMELE.COM/2-7**

Brushing Video

SAY THIS

Followers, today we would like you to share your tactic to making brushing enjoyable for your kids or yourself! Watch how these little ones do it!

,,

DESCRIPTION

Make brushing fun! Do your viewers have their own suggestions?

LINK: **WWW.RACHELMELE.COM/2-8**

National Toothache Day

SAY THIS

Today is National Toothache Day. To prevent a toothache, try these tips: 1) Routine dental visits. 2) Avoid sugary foods. 3) Avoid acidic drinks. 4) Brush at least two times a day. 5) Floss daily. If you have a toothache, be sure to give us a call – we can help!

99

DESCRIPTION

Provide tips for your followers to avoid toothaches.

LINK: **WWW.RACHELMELE.COM/2-9**

Valentine's Day Dental Humor

SAY THIS

The Beatles said, "all you need is love." We say all you need is love AND floss. What are your plans for Valentine's Day?

,,

DESCRIPTION

Include a graphic of a toothbrush and a heart. Remember to respond to all comments you receive.

LINK: **WWW.RACHELMELE.COM/2-10**

Patient's After Photos

SAY THIS

Meet our patient [patient's name] who received Zoom Whitening. Don't you think [his/her] results look wonderful? This could be you! Call to find out more information about Zoom Whitening today!

”

DESCRIPTION

Take a picture of patient with this or another teeth whitening procedure.

LINK: WWW.RACHELMELE.COM/ 2-11

How to Brush

SAY THIS

Moms & Dads! Watch this helpful video on how to teach your child to brush their teeth. Don't forget to stay on track with their bi-annual cleanings at [Practice Name]! Give us a call, at [Practice Phone #], if you have any questions.

,,

DESCRIPTION

Include the phone number to the practice and link to video or create your own video.

LINK: **WWW.RACHELMELE.COM/2-12**

Dental Fun

SAY THIS

It has been said that the average woman smiles approximately 62 times a day compared to men who only smile 8 times a day. Tomorrow is Valentine's Day. Guys, don't forget to smile at your lady.

,,

DESCRIPTION

Valentine's Day is a great excuse to engage with your patients on social media. Get creative about the photo you include with this post. One idea is to take a photo of a man frowning next to a women smiling from ear to ear.

LINK: **WWW.RACHELMELE.COM/ 2-13**

Valentine's Day

SAY THIS

Nothing says Happy Valentine's Day like a tooth ring for your special somebody. Tag someone who would love this!

,,

DESCRIPTION

Suggest dental and Valentines related gifts like this one to your patients.

LINK: **WWW.RACHELMELE.COM/2-14**

Patient Testimonial

SAY THIS

A fabulous testimonial from one of our patients, [Patient Name] on [his/ her] Invisalign treatment! Find out how you can achieve straighter and healthier teeth without braces. Call or check out our website for more information!

"

DESCRIPTION

Take a video of one of your patients with a success story on a product! Make sure to tag them.

LINK: **WWW.RACHELMELE.COM/2-15**

Children's Book Drive

SAY THIS

Got Books? Don't know what to do with your gently used children's books? Bring them to [Practice Name]! Now until March 16th, we are hosting a children's book drive. All books will be donated to [Donation Location] on March 18th.

"

DESCRIPTION

Capture a photo of a team member holding a book and write all the book drive info on the picture. Book donations could be taken to a local library!

LINK: **WWW.RACHELMELE.COM/2-16**

Random Acts of Kindness

SAY THIS

It's Random Acts of Kindness Day. [Doctor Name] volunteers every year at [name location]. What random acts of kindness have you done or experienced?

99

DESCRIPTION

Take a video of doctor describing his/her random act of kindness. Be sure to respond to posts!

LINK: **WWW.RACHELMELE.COM/2-17**

Friday Night Contest

SAY THIS

It's Friday; movie night is on us. First person to comment on this post gets two tickets to the movies and a $50 gift card to [Restaurant Name]. [Link to a local restaurant]

"

DESCRIPTION

Be sure to keep it local. Posts like this will keep your followers checking your site.

LINK: **WWW.RACHELMELE.COM/2-18**

Smile

SAY THIS

What makes you smile?

,,

DESCRIPTION

Capture a photo of a patient smiling to
add to post. Feature a patient with a
great smile and their reason to smile!
Don't forget to tag them!

LINK: **WWW.RACHELMELE.COM/2-19**

Ice Cream

SAY THIS

Our staff is treating themselves to ice cream.

Thanks to [Practice Doctor(s)]!

"

DESCRIPTION

Anytime your practice enjoys a treat as a team, be sure to post about it with a picture.

LINK: **WWW.RACHELMELE.COM/2-20**

President's Day

SAY THIS

Happy President's Day. President Washington performed his own teeth extractions. Glad our patients know better!

99

DESCRIPTION

This post could get really fun with a picture of a team member dressed up.

LINK: WWW.RACHELMELE.COM/2-21

Children's Dental Health Month

SAY THIS

Celebrate National Children's Dental Health Month in February by printing these activity pages for your kids and their friends!

,,

DESCRIPTION

Promote National Children's Dental Health Month by implementing their campaign resources into your practice, including posters, print-outs and more.

LINK: **WWW.RACHELMELE.COM/2-22**

Dental Tip

SAY THIS

To avoid having bad breath, [Practice Name] has a tip of the day for our Facebook Fans: Leave a toothbrush at work in your desk so you can brush your teeth after lunch.

"

DESCRIPTION

Provide tips for your followers
to avoid having bad breath.

LINK: **WWW.RACHELMELE.COM/ 2-23**

Patient Feature

SAY THIS

We recently treated [Patient Name] for [procedure]. This is what they had to say. [Patient commentary on procedure].

,,

DESCRIPTION

Featuring your patients on posts can increase the popularity of the post as it can be shared by the patient and reach a larger audience.

LINK: WWW.RACHELMELE.COM/2-24

Brush to Music

SAY THIS

Who says brushing your teeth is boring? Pump up the volume and brush with these fun beats to play while you brush. Public Service Announcement: music may cause sudden dancing and giggles in children and adults.

,,

DESCRIPTION

Link to a blog with your recommendations for teeth brushing songs or even better get the whole team to brush to your favorite song on video.

LINK: **WWW.RACHELMELE.COM/ 2-25**

Dentist in Action

SAY THIS

Catch [Doctor(s) Name(s)] in action with our patient [Patient Name]. Call to make your appointment today at [Practice Name]! [Practice Phone Number]

,,

DESCRIPTION

Capture a photo of your dentist and patient during their appointment to add to post. Be sure to get written permission.

LINK: **WWW.RACHELMELE.COM/2-26**

Floss Before a Date

SAY THIS

Did you know, three in four people are more likely to floss only before a big event? Are you more likely to floss before a first date, interview or some other big event? Read more about how often adults floss.

99

DESCRIPTION

Ask your followers a question regarding their dental habits to open the door to conversation. Make sure you respond to their answers!

LINK: **WWW.RACHELMELE.COM/2-27**

Apples & Saliva

SAY THIS

The high water content in apples helps stimulate the flow of saliva. This protects against decay by washing away food particles and buffering acid! Click "Like" if you love apples! What's your favorite type?

"

DESCRIPTION

Share this fact about apples with your followers and get them involved by asking a question!

LINK: **WWW.RACHELMELE.COM/2-28**

Leap Year Patient Fun

SAY THIS

[Patient Name] is a Leap Year baby. Technically [he/she] is only [X] years old. Do you know anyone else that is born on Leap Year?

"

DESCRIPTION

Take a picture with your team blowing out candles for this patient. Get your patient's permission for this posting.

LINK: **WWW.RACHELMELE.COM/2-29**

Yellow Teeth

SAY THIS

Are you wondering what turns your teeth

yellow? Take a guess... then read this.

"

DESCRIPTION

Add link to post or write your own blog

post on factors that turn your teeth yellow.

LINK: **WWW.RACHELMELE.COM/3-1**

Dr. Seuss' B-Day

SAY THIS

Happy Birthday Dr. Seuss! Check out how [Practice Name] is celebrating Read Across America today!

99

DESCRIPTION

Capture a photo of team members reading a Dr. Seuss book, and even dressed up as him, too!

LINK: **WWW.RACHELMELE.COM/3-2**

Employee Appreciation Day

SAY THIS

*Today is Employee Appreciation Day!
We want to thank our amazing team for bringing
their best to our practice every day! What do you
love about our team? Let us know and we will
share your comments during our team lunch.*

" "

DESCRIPTION

Dedicate this post to your team! Whether it's a
group picture or individual photos, they are in
the spotlight today! Make sure you tag them.

LINK: **WWW.RACHELMELE.COM/3-3**

2x2

SAY THIS

Did you know that the bacteria that causes cavities is contagious? It's true! The bacteria can be passed through your saliva. Don't forget to floss & brush 2x a day for 2 minutes to get those sugar bugs out!

"

DESCRIPTION

Find interesting ways to educate your patients on a variety of topics they might find interesting.

LINK: **WWW.RACHELMELE.COM/3-4**

National Oreo Cookie Day

SAY THIS

Happy National Oreo Cookie Day!
Guess what our staff is having for
lunch today?

99

DESCRIPTION

Have fun with your posts. Include a
picture or video of the team eating Oreos.

LINK: WWW.RACHELMELE.COM/3-5

National Dentist Day

SAY THIS

Happy NATIONAL DENTIST DAY - Thank you to all of our mouth heroes who work hard every day! Leave a comment telling us why YOU love YOUR dentist.

"

DESCRIPTION

Dedicate this post to your dentists! Share their photo with kind words and promote follower involvement by having them tag their dentists.

LINK: WWW.RACHELMELE.COM/3-6

Question

SAY THIS

Guess which of our team member's smile this is?

99

DESCRIPTION

Take a picture of a team member's smile and post it. Encourage followers to be part of the online guessing game.

LINK: **WWW.RACHELMELE.COM/3-7**

St. Patrick's Day Approaching

SAY THIS

St. Patrick's Day is around the corner, and you want to be wearing this shirt! -SAFETY FIRST DRINK WITH A DENTIST- Order now!

"

DESCRIPTION

Display links to products related to dentistry that your followers could purchase or get a good laugh from!

LINK: WWW.RACHELMELE.COM/3-8

Question

SAY THIS

How good is your Dental IQ? Take this

short quiz and tell us your score.

"

DESCRIPTION

Post the answers to the quiz.

LINK: **WWW.RACHELMELE.COM/3-9**

Child's First Visit

SAY THIS

FIRST BIRTHDAY = FIRST DENTIST VISIT - It's important to schedule your child's first dental visit at [Practice Name] by their first birthday. Read more for what to expect on their first visit!

,,

DESCRIPTION

Add link to or write your own blog post about when children should be seen by a dentist.

LINK: **WWW.RACHELMELE.COM/3-10**

Dental Fun

SAY THIS

The term "indentured servant" has a story behind it. In the colonial days, debtors were shipped from Europe to America to work as servants. Instead of signing a contract, they sealed their agreement by leaving their dental imprint in wax. Cool right?

"

DESCRIPTION

Link the definition of "indentured servant" to the post.

LINK: **WWW.RACHELMELE.COM/3-11**

Quote

SAY THIS

"Start every day with a smile and get it over with."

~W.C. Fields

,,

DESCRIPTION

Get a picture of your doctor or a staff member just waking up with messy hair, PJs, no make-up but the BIGGEST smile ever.

LINK: WWW.RACHELMELE.COM/3-12

Daylight Saving

SAY THIS

It's daylight saving time! Use this survival guide to make this day easier and don't forget to fix your clocks so you don't miss your appointment!

,,

DESCRIPTION

Remind your followers to set their clocks at the right time so they don't miss their appointments!

LINK: **WWW.RACHELMELE.COM/3-13**

Pi Day

SAY THIS

Happy Pi Day from
[Practice Name]!

,,

DESCRIPTION

Include a picture of a pie and the pi sign.

LINK: **WWW.RACHELMELE.COM/3-14**

Backwards Day

SAY THIS

Today is Backwards Day at [Practice Name]. Catch our team and our office completely BACKWARDS!

99

DESCRIPTION

Turn everything backwards! The office and uniforms! Make sure to take pictures of all the backwards fun and add them with your post!

LINK: **WWW.RACHELMELE.COM/3-15**

Blog Post

SAY THIS

*Bridges & Crowns... no, we are not talking about a
road trip to see the Queen! Learn more about
DENTAL bridges and crowns here.*

"

DESCRIPTION

Add a link to a blog post all
about crowns and bridges.

LINK: **WWW.RACHELMELE.COM/3-16**

St. Patrick's Day

SAY THIS

Happy Saint Patrick's Day! Things to watch out for: The food coloring used in green beer can penetrate your teeth, resulting in a green smile. You might want to hold the mustard, too. If you can't resist green beer or mustard, give us a call at [Practice Phone #].

,,

DESCRIPTION

Dentists are pretty busy after this holiday due to these reasons listed above. Provide a link to this article explaining why.

LINK: **WWW.RACHELMELE.COM/3-17**

Contest

SAY THIS

MARCH CONTEST! If you "Check In" at our office on Facebook, you will be entered to win a [Prize].

,,

DESCRIPTION

Create an incentive for followers to check in when at your practice by giving away a gift card. Be sure you know your state's rules about giving gifts to patients.

LINK: WWW.RACHELMELE.COM/3-18

Dental Anxiety

SAY THIS

Do you have dental anxiety? You aren't alone. WebMD shares tips to help you feel less nervous.

„

DESCRIPTION

Write a blog post about dental anxiety. Blogging has a significant impact on your search results.

LINK: WWW.RACHELMELE.COM/3-19

First Day of Spring

SAY THIS

Happy First Day of Spring! How are you going to be celebrating spring today? Going to the park? A picnic lunch? Let us know. Enjoy the day!

"

DESCRIPTION

Capture a picture of the outside of your practice displaying the sun shinning and colorful flowers! Respond to posts.

LINK: **WWW.RACHELMELE.COM/3-20**

DIY-Whitening Methods

SAY THIS

Please consult our practice prior to attempting any DIY methods of at-home whitening or dental care! Give us a call with any questions!

99

DESCRIPTION

You are the ultimate resource on best practices for teeth whitening. Your patients want to know various ways to whiten. Educate them.

LINK: **WWW.RACHELMELE.COM/3-21**

Father of Dentistry

SAY THIS

Happy Birthday Pierre Fauchard, the father of modern dentistry! Get to know a little more about him!

99

DESCRIPTION

Include a link to an article about Pierre Fauchard, or write about him yourself and post it on your blog.

LINK: WWW.RACHELMELE.COM/3-22

Dental Check Ups

SAY THIS

Regular dental checkups for kids are not important...
SAID NO ONE EVER! Read this article to understand
the importance of regular checkups for kids!

"

DESCRIPTION

Provide your followers with an article
explaining why regular checkups are still
important even if their child still has
their baby teeth. Write your own blog
post or link to an article.

LINK: **WWW.RACHELMELE.COM/3-23**

Video

SAY THIS

This video is too cute. Kids say the funniest things. "David after the Dentist"

,,

DESCRIPTION

This is the kind of post that patients will "share" and your office will get more exposure.

LINK: **WWW.RACHELMELE.COM/3-24**

Pregnancy & Dental

SAY THIS

Are you pregnant? Take care of you and your baby, and [Practice Name] will take care of your teeth! Keep reading to find out more information on dental care during pregnancy!

99

DESCRIPTION

Rich content about a variety of topics can help your website and social presence get found online. Write about as many topics as possible.

LINK: **WWW.RACHELMELE.COM/3-25**

Silly Hat Day

SAY THIS

It's Silly Hat Day. Catch our [Patient(s) First Name(s)] rocking [his/her] [hat description] for Silly Hat Day! Post a picture in the comments of your silly hat.

,,

DESCRIPTION

Make sure you photograph all patients wearing a silly hat. Have some silly hats on hand in the office to share for photos.

LINK: **WWW.RACHELMELE.COM/3-26**

Mustache Day

SAY THIS

Mustache you a question? Today is Mustache Day at [Practice Name]! Take a look at our patients who rocked the stache!

,,

DESCRIPTION

Leading up to this day, get pictures of patients with mustaches. Add pictures to your post and don't forget to tag them!

LINK: **WWW.RACHELMELE.COM/3-27**

Oral Cancer Prevention

SAY THIS

Oral Cancer KILLS as many people as melanoma and is now more common than leukemia.

"

DESCRIPTION

Make your followers aware of the consequences of ignoring symptoms.

LINK: **WWW.RACHELMELE.COM/3-28**

Dental Fun

SAY THIS

Here is a fun dental fact! In Medieval Germany, the only cure for a toothache was to kiss a donkey.

Pucker up!

,,

DESCRIPTION

Search for picture of a donkey on istockphoto.com or another photo site to add to your post.

LINK: **WWW.RACHELMELE.COM/3-29**

Gum Disease

SAY THIS

Pregnant women with gum (periodontal) disease could be at risk of having their babies born early or small. If you are pregnant, be sure to schedule regular periodontal checkups.

,,

DESCRIPTION

Anyone pregnant in your office?
Include a photo of them taking care of
their teeth or write a blog post.

LINK: **WWW.RACHELMELE.COM/3-30**

How to Floss Video

SAY THIS

Just in case you forgot, here is a reminder!
Watch this video to see how to properly
floss your teeth.

,,

DESCRIPTION

Ask different people in your office
to show each step of the flossing
process in a video.

LINK: **WWW.RACHELMELE.COM/3-31**

April Fool's Day

SAY THIS

April Fool's Day is a great day to share some fun dental facts.

99

DESCRIPTION

Find your own fun dental facts to share or share these in the link below.

LINK: **WWW.RACHELMELE.COM/4-1**

Children's Book Day

SAY THIS

It's Children's Book Day. Our office has more than [#of children's books] children's books, from "The Cat and the Hat" to "Goodnight Moon." We also have "Arthur's Loose Tooth" and "The Berenstain Bears Visit the Dentist." Feel free to borrow one and teach your kids good dental health.

"

DESCRIPTION

Make sure to take a picture of all the available books.

LINK: **WWW.RACHELMELE.COM/4-2**

Facial Protection Month

April is National Facial Protection Month. Did you know that sports accidents account for up to 39% of dental injuries in children? Always have your kids wear a mouth guard! Ask us about the custom-fit mouth guards that we offer!

"

Patient awareness can benefit your patients.

LINK: WWW.RACHELMELE.COM/4-3

Patient Referral

SAY THIS

32% of Americans cite bad breath as the least attractive trait of their co-workers. Do you know a co-worker with bad breath? Give them a [Practice Name] referral card and if they become a patient, we would like to thank you at your next visit.

,,

DESCRIPTION

Make sure to keep track of patients who participate in promotions.

LINK: **WWW.RACHELMELE.COM/4-4**

Oral Cancer Awareness

SAY THIS

April is Oral Cancer Awareness Month. Call our office at [Practice Phone Number] to schedule an oral cancer screening. A VELscope screening takes less than a minute and detects abnormalities.

,,

DESCRIPTION

Link a video of your practice conducting a screening using VELscope and add it to this post.

LINK: **WWW.RACHELMELE.COM/4-5**

Bad Breath

SAY THIS

Does your child have bad breath? Find out five surprising reasons for bad breath in children! Keep reading!

99

DESCRIPTION

Write a blog post about bad breath for children or link to this post below.

LINK: WWW.RACHELMELE.COM/4-6

Toothbrushing Song

SAY THIS

A video to entertain your day: watch

"The Tooth Brushing Song."

by Tebo The Tooth

"

DESCRIPTION

Share this fun video or make your own.

LINK: WWW.RACHELMELE.COM/4-7

Schedule Opening

SAY THIS

Are you due for a cleaning?

We have a few openings this week.

Call us at [Practice Phone #]

to see if one might work for you.

"

DESCRIPTION

You might want to add a cell phone number and post it on your page as well. Texting is a great way to communicate.

LINK: WWW.RACHELMELE.COM/4-8

Smile

SAY THIS

Believe it or not, smiling boosts your immune system! Here are some other interesting facts about smiling:

,,

DESCRIPTION

Create a 20 second video of each person in the practice smiling and put the video to music.

LINK: **WWW.RACHELMELE.COM/4-9**

Dental Couponer

Are you a COUPONER? If so, we want to see pictures of your stocked up toothpaste/toothbrushes.

"

DESCRIPTION

You may be surprised to learn how many of your patients have stock piles of toothpaste and toothbrushes from all their good couponing habits.

LINK: WWW.RACHELMELE.COM/4-10

Video

SAY THIS

Have you ever wondered, "what if kids were dentists?" Well here it is! Tell us what you think.

,,

DESCRIPTION

Include a link to this video or create your own video. Don't forget to comment back to followers.

LINK: **WWW.RACHELMELE.COM/4-11**

Forgotten Toothpaste

SAY THIS

OH NO, NO TOOTHPASTE.....What to do when you've run out or forgotten your toothpaste?!

"

DESCRIPTION

These are common issues patient deal with. Ask them to comment on what they do when they run out of toothpaste.

LINK: WWW.RACHELMELE.COM/4-12

Braces Care

SAY THIS

Not sure how to brush or floss while wearing traditional braces? Check out this helpful video; soon you'll be brushing & flossing like a pro! Questions about orthodontic treatment? Give us a call to set up a complimentary orthodontic consultation for your child or yourself:

[Practice Phone Number]

,,

DESCRIPTION

Link this video to your post or make one on your own with your team members.

LINK: **WWW.RACHELMELE.COM/4-13**

April Break

SAY THIS

Need to make an appointment for your kids while on April break? No problem! [Practice Name] is offering more appointments for your convenience. Contact the office to schedule an appointment today -[Practice Phone #].

The schedule is filling fast!

"

DESCRIPTION

Be sure to have some appointment openings quickly available for callers.

LINK: **WWW.RACHELMELE.COM/4-14**

Tax Day

SAY THIS

Tax Day, need we say more? Come in to the office today from [Time Slot] for a free toothbrush! Brush, brush, brush taxes away!

,,

DESCRIPTION

Arrange 4-5 hours where patients can come in to receive a complementry tooth brush! Take a picture of the toothbrush you are giving away to post.

LINK: **WWW.RACHELMELE.COM/4-15**

Dental Pet Care

SAY THIS

Even your pet needs dental care. Don't forget to take your pet to the veterinarian for a dental exam. Begin a dental care regimen and schedule regular checkups.

,,

DESCRIPTION

Link picture to post of team member with dog. Make it funny. Or if you have a relationship with a local veterinarian, include a link to their website.

LINK: WWW.RACHELMELE.COM/4-16

Reminder

SAY THIS

Wait a second! Has it been over 6 months since

we've seen your smile? That won't do...Call us

ASAP. We'll have you in and out quick

– and your mouth will thank you!

[Practice Phone #]

"

DESCRIPTION

Consider creating a video with your

doctor saying this post and include the

words as captions.

LINK: WWW.RACHELMELE.COM/4-17

What's the Name of that Song?

SAY THIS

[Patient Name] was captured on video humming a song while being worked on... Can you guess the song?

99

DESCRIPTION

Capture on video a patient willing to hum a part of the song for followers to guess!

LINK: WWW.RACHELMELE.COM/4-18

Patient Video

SAY THIS

Would you like to be the face of [Practice Name]? We're producing a new TV commercial, and we are looking for a patient to be the face of our practice. Just submit a video on our Facebook page telling us why you'd be the best face of our practice. Videos must be received before August 1.

,,

DESCRIPTION

If you have ever considered creating a TV commercial, get your patients involved.

LINK: **WWW.RACHELMELE.COM/4-19**

Bleaching

SAY THIS

Attention Parents! Bleaching your kid's teeth before they are fully developed can lead to problems.

,,

DESCRIPTION

This important information could be beneficial to your patients. Blog about it.

LINK: **WWW.RACHELMELE.COM/4-20**

Look-alike Day

SAY THIS

In honor of National Look-alike Day, we made this collage of our dentist and the celebrities we think they look the most like!

What do you think?

99

DESCRIPTION

This is a fun post! Take full advantage and make your followers laugh!

LINK: **WWW.RACHELMELE.COM/4-21**

Early Earth Day Tip

SAY THIS

An early Earth Day tip – conserve water by turning off the faucet while brushing your teeth! What other tips can you share?

99

DESCRIPTION

Get input from other team members on what you can present to your followers on Earth Day.

LINK: WWW.RACHELMELE.COM/4-22

Earth Day

SAY THIS

Happy Earth Day! [Doctor(s) Name(s)] celebrated Earth Day by planting a "Dentist-Tree"! Join us in beautifying our planet. Stop by our office between [Hours] and pick up a packet of wildflower seeds as our gift to you and the environment. (While supplies last).

"

DESCRIPTION

Buy a small tree and plant it. Make sure to document it with pictures that you can add to your post. Buy a packet of wild- flower seeds to give away to your patients!

LINK: **WWW.RACHELMELE.COM/4-23**

Invisalign®
Tip

SAY THIS

Attention Invisalign® Users!

*Remember when cleaning your Invisalign®
aligners, never use hot water as this may cause
irreparable warping of the plastic.*

,,

DESCRIPTION

Give followers tips on certain products or
services you provide at your dental
practice. This can also be a good way to
advertise your products and services.

LINK: WWW.RACHELMELE.COM/4-24

Question

SAY THIS

When was your last cleaning and checkup? If it has been more than 6 months, give us a call! [Telephone #].

"

DESCRIPTION

Make sure you add the phone number and link to the practice website.

LINK: WWW.RACHELMELE.COM/4-25

Spring Dental Fun

SAY THIS

If April showers bring May flowers, we should be seeing smiles blooming soon!

,,

DESCRIPTION

Post picture of the blooming flowers around your office.

LINK: **WWW.RACHELMELE.COM/4-26**

True or False

SAY THIS

True or False: The combination of crushed strawberries and baking soda as a homemade teeth whitening remedy can help remove stains? Comment your answers!

"

DESCRIPTION

Quiz Time! Leave your followers some time to guess and comment their answers! Toward the end of the day post the answer with some words of advice!

LINK: WWW.RACHELMELE.COM/4-27

Dental Fun

SAY THIS

Some dental humor for this beautiful day!

"

DESCRIPTION

Share a comic strip like the example below. Remember not to upload the image as your own if it doesn't belong to you. Sharing is ok.

LINK: WWW.RACHELMELE.COM/4-28

Administrative Professionals Day

SAY THIS

Happy Administrative Professionals Day to our amazing Administrators at [Practice Name]! Our practice could not run without you. Thank you for all that you do!

,,

DESCRIPTION

Add pictures to your post and don't forget to tag them!

LINK: WWW.RACHELMELE.COM/4-29

Teeth, Eyes, or Hair?

SAY THIS

Would you rather have: perfect teeth, perfect eyesight or perfect hair? According to Glamour Beauty, 44% say teeth.

99

DESCRIPTION

Link to this website page.

LINK: **WWW.RACHELMELE.COM/4-30**

Child Anxiety

SAY THIS

Is your child afraid to come see us? Here's an article from WebMD about easing your child's fear of the dentist.

99

DESCRIPTION

Link picture to post.

LINK: **WWW.RACHELMELE.COM/5-1**

Baseball Giveaway!

SAY THIS

Baseball season is upon us – enter to win this game day goodie basket! Comment your favorite team below and share this post to win this basket filled with baseball goodies! The shared post with the most likes will be the selected winner! [Insert Picture of basket]

"

DESCRIPTION

Go to the closest grocery store and gather up some goodies! Sunglasses, energy drinks, nuts, popcorn, and some Big League Chew. Throw them in a basket, and now you have a contest prize! Check out this example below!

LINK: **WWW.RACHELMELE.COM/5-2**

Electric Toothbrush

SAY THIS

Do you know how to brush with an electric toothbrush? You may be surprised! Keep reading and find out more.

,,

DESCRIPTION

Put together a quick video explaining how to properly use an electric toothbrush to go along with this post.

LINK: **WWW.RACHELMELE.COM/5-3**

Video

SAY THIS

Check out this video from Crest® as a blogger discusses the importance of having a brighter, whiter smile just in time for life's important and unexpected moments.

,,

DESCRIPTION

Include the link below in your posts.

LINK: WWW.RACHELMELE.COM/5-4

Cinco de Mayo

SAY THIS

Happy Cinco de Mayo! Or Cinco de Clean Teeth.
Ponchos and Sombreros for everyone! Check
out our cool patients who let us dress them up!

"

DESCRIPTION

Get a sombrero and poncho then have your
patients wear them for a silly Cinco de Mayo
picture! Do a picture collage and get all
your patients involved today.

LINK: **WWW.RACHELMELE.COM/5-5**

Baseball
Spirit Day

---- SAY THIS ----

Play Ball! Yesterday we celebrated our monthly
Spirit Day - Baseball themed! Whether Red Sox,
Yankees or Mets fans at [Practice Name] we love
to have fun!

,,

---- DESCRIPTION ----

Add pictures to your post and don't forget
to tag team members!

LINK: **WWW.RACHELMELE.COM/5-6**

Toothpaste Usage

SAY THIS

Over the years our patients have shared the many other ways they use toothpaste. Here are some of our favorites.

,,

DESCRIPTION

Write a blog about all the ways other ways patients have told you they use toothpaste. Like zapping zits and cleaning headlights.

LINK: WWW.RACHELMELE.COM/5-7

Team Appreciation

SAY THIS

Today we are featuring our Team Member of the Month, [Team Member Name], our [Practice Position/Title]. [Team Member Name] ensures our patients are fully informed about their dental care by answering any questions they may have. Thanks, [Team Member Name]!

,,

DESCRIPTION

Display your team members on social media by saying great things about them! Look at what this practice said about their team member of the month!

LINK: **WWW.RACHELMELE.COM/5-8**

Graduation is Near

SAY THIS

It's graduation time. Time to start looking for a job? Need interview tips? Find them here! Feel free to tag someone who could benefit from these tips!

99

DESCRIPTION

Recent graduates will appreciate this post! Share this article below or write your own blog post sharing interview and career advice for soon to be dental graduates!

LINK: **WWW.RACHELMELE.COM/5-9**

Team Member Anniversary

SAY THIS

Happy Anniversary to our team member,

[Team Member Name].

Thank you for being a great addition to our

dental family!

"

DESCRIPTION

Celebrate when your team hits a milestone anniversary by posting pictures and videos of the celebration.

LINK: **WWW.RACHELMELE.COM/5-10**

Toothbrush Storage

SAY THIS

[Practice Name] recommends that a toothbrush is kept at least six feet away from a toilet to avoid airborne particles resulting from the flush.

Where do you keep your toothbrush?

DESCRIPTION

Take a picture of a toothbrush sitting on a toilet. Yuck!

LINK: **WWW.RACHELMELE.COM/5-11**

Quote

SAY THIS

"You are never fully dressed

until you wear a smile."

~Martin Charnin

,,

DESCRIPTION

Post a picture of the doctor in his/her

PJs with a frown next to a picture of the

doctor fully dressed with a smile from

ear to ear.

LINK: **WWW.RACHELMELE.COM/5-12**

Dental Fun

SAY THIS

Cotton Candy is our toothpaste flavor of the month! What is your favorite toothpaste flavor?

"

DESCRIPTION

Include a picture of cotton candy toothpaste. Encourage your followers to post comments and be sure to reply to their comments.

LINK: WWW.RACHELMELE.COM/5-13

Mouthwash

SAY THIS

Who here uses mouthwash after brushing their teeth? Prove it. Post your mouthwash photos/videos here.

,,

DESCRIPTION

Post a video of the doctor or a team member using mouthwash.

LINK: WWW.RACHELMELE.COM/5-14

Cheek Challenge

SAY THIS

Cheek retractor challenge! A new Cheek Retractor Challenge inspired by the game Speak Out. Check our team out – this was too much fun!

,,

DESCRIPTION

Pull out your cheek retractors and take a video of your team trying to talk with them in or play the official "Speak Out" board game.

LINK: WWW.RACHELMELE.COM/5-15

Office Map

SAY THIS

Just in case you didn't know, here is the map showing our location(s)! Now click on the map and make your way down to our office!

"

DESCRIPTION

Add Google maps location to the post.

LINK: **WWW.RACHELMELE.COM/5-16**

Question

SAY THIS

Another great review! What do YOU like best about being a patient at [Practice Name]?

99

DESCRIPTION

Link a recent patient review or ask a patient to leave a review before they leave their appointment.

LINK: WWW.RACHELMELE.COM/5-17

Dental Fun

SAY THIS

This is how we feel when patients can't decide which fluoride flavor they want!

"

DESCRIPTION

Add meme / graphic to your post.

LINK: WWW.RACHELMELE.COM/5-18

Pre-Memorial Day Promotion

SAY THIS

Memorial Day is not the only day we support our Troops. You are always remembered and we are always thankful! Tag a veteran you are thankful for!

"

DESCRIPTION

Make sure you respond and give thanks to veterans tagged on post.

LINK: WWW.RACHELMELE.COM/5-19

Nail Biting

SAY THIS

Nail biting is generally triggered by stress and most often decreases with age. That being said, nail biting is unsanitary, unattractive, as well as unhealthy for your teeth! Stop today! Don't believe us? Read this!

"

DESCRIPTION

Keep your followers informed on articles of interest.

LINK: **WWW.RACHELMELE.COM/5-20**

Summer Reminder

SAY THIS

Just in time for summer!

[Practice Name] is open [#of days] days a week!

Schedule your child today!

Appointments are filling up fast this summer!

99

DESCRIPTION

Be sure to let your patients know when your office hours change during different seasons.

LINK: WWW.RACHELMELE.COM/5-21

Brushing Calendar

SAY THIS

Parents! Summer is approaching – brushing can be tough on a summer schedule. Use this fun calendar to keep your kids on track. Feel free to use stickers or fun colored markers to check off brushing and flossing twice each day!

"

DESCRIPTION

Add link to printable calendar.

LINK: **WWW.RACHELMELE.COM/5-22**

Tips for Graduates!

SAY THIS

From dentist to graduate – you will want to read this! Tag someone who recently has or is getting ready to graduate.

„

DESCRIPTION

Write your own dental blog post on

tips for recent or future graduates or

share the link below!

LINK: WWW.RACHELMELE.COM/5-23

True or False

True or False: Can the sun lighten your teeth?

,,

DESCRIPTION

(FALSE)

Quiz Time! Leave your followers some time to guess and comment on their answers! Towards the end of the day post the answer with some words of advice or a link to this article!

LINK: **WWW.RACHELMELE.COM/5-24**

Mom & Dad

SAY THIS

Mom & Dad - [Practice Name] offers adult orthodontics! Call to schedule your complimentary orthodontic consultation today!

"

DESCRIPTION

Promote the varied procedures that the practice provides.

LINK: WWW.RACHELMELE.COM/5-25

Business Appreciation

SAY THIS

Congratulations to [Business Name] on opening their new store at [Location]. Can't wait to stop by and check things out!

"

DESCRIPTION

It is great to show appreciation to

other businesses – plus it gives

your business a great reputation.

LINK: WWW.RACHELMELE.COM/5-26

Show Us Your Smile Contest!

SAY THIS

Enter our Show us your

Summer Selfie Smile Contest!

Don't forget to post a fun family picture to our

FB page & you'll be entered to win [Prize].

"

DESCRIPTION

Make sure to include all rules to the contest!
Include start, end time and voting process and
post the winners when complete.

LINK: **WWW.RACHELMELE.COM/5-27**

Memorial Day

SAY THIS

*In honor of Memorial Day, our family at
[Practice Name] accepted the 22 push up
challenge! We want to send out a big thank you
to all of those men and women who have served
our wonderful country! We are forever grateful
for your past and continued services to protect
us and our homeland. Thank you!*

"

DESCRIPTION

Gather your dental crew, set up your camera
and PUSH UP! This is a fun but respectful
way to show gratitude to those who served
our country and entertain your followers!

LINK: **WWW.RACHELMELE.COM/5-28**

Patient Feature

SAY THIS

Congratulations to our [Patient Name] who is going to prom. Look at that beautiful smile! Is your prom smile ready?

,,

DESCRIPTION

Feature a recent patient who is attending prom! Make sure you tag them in this post and ask them to repost/share!

LINK: WWW.RACHELMELE.COM/5-29

Quote

SAY THIS

"A smile can brighten the darkest day."

~Author Unknown

99

DESCRIPTION

Pick a day that is really cloudy out. Post a picture along with this quote of a team member smiling from ear to ear with the dark clouds in the background.

LINK: **WWW.RACHELMELE.COM/5-30**

World No Tobacco Day

SAY THIS

It's World No Tobacco Day and we would like you to just say "no." Tobacco causes stinky breath, stained teeth, bone loss, shrinking gums, mouth sores, decreased sense of taste and smell, and a poorly healing mouth. Do we need to say more? Check out this video:

"

DESCRIPTION

Inform your followers about the dental harm of smoking tobacco on World No Tobacco Day! Share a video or make one of your own listing the reasons why one should never smoke!

LINK: **WWW.RACHELMELE.COM/5-31**

Comment Below

SAY THIS

HELLO FOLLOWERS!

Comment below your best / most ridiculous/ no-sense-making excuse to reschedule or cancel your dentist appointment! No worries, we won't judge!

,,

DESCRIPTION

Show your followers your great sense of humor! Make sure you comment back on their posts and post an excuse of your own, too!

LINK: **WWW.RACHELMELE.COM/6-1**

Repeat Day

SAY THIS

Call your dentist. I said, "Call your dentist."
(It's National Repeat Day).
[Practice Phone #], [Practice Phone #].

""

DESCRIPTION

Witty posts are needed to

get a smile out of your followers!

LINK: **WWW.RACHELMELE.COM/6-2**

Teeth Whitening

SAY THIS

If only my teeth were as white as my legs.

"

DESCRIPTION

Take a photo of someone's white (pre-summer tan) legs next to a picture of stained teeth. Or use an example like the link below.

LINK: **WWW.RACHELMELE.COM/6-3**

Game

SAY THIS

Our staff is obsessed with this fun game called "Match Three Dental." How high of a score can you get?

"

DESCRIPTION

Share a picture or video of your staff having a blast playing this game. Show your followers that fun and games also happen at the office! Include a link to the game, too.

LINK: **WWW.RACHELMELE.COM/6-4**

Summer Drawing Contest

SAY THIS

Hey Kids! Draw us a picture of your favorite thing to do in the summer, for a chance to win a $25 gift card. All drawings will be displayed in our office and patients will vote for their favorite drawing! Hand in your drawings by the end of the week and then voting begins! Winner will be chosen by the end of the month!

DESCRIPTION

Make sure you are clear with rules to the contest.

LINK: WWW.RACHELMELE.COM/6-5

Read To Patients

SAY THIS

We caught [Team Member Name] reading a book to one of our little patients, [Patient Name]. What's your kiddos favorite book to read?

"

DESCRIPTION

Highlight the little things that happen in the office each day by capturing it on photo, video, or even Live.

LINK: **WWW.RACHELMELE.COM/6-6**

Best Friend Day

SAY THIS

Would they hold your hand while you get your wisdom teeth pulled or never let you miss a dental appointment? That's a true friend! National Best Friend Day - Tag your best friend!

,,

DESCRIPTION

Create a collage of photos with each team member's best friend and post why they've been friends for so long.

LINK: WWW.RACHELMELE.COM/6-7

Mouth Guard

SAY THIS

Visit our blog to learn how to take care of your teeth while playing sports by using a mouth guard, properly caring for a knocked out tooth and avoiding injury to your mouth. Tag an athlete that could benefit from these tips

,,

DESCRIPTION

Write your own dental blog post featuring the tips and tricks of teeth care while playing sports!

LINK: **WWW.RACHELMELE.COM/6-8**

Damaging Foods

SAY THIS

What are summer's most tooth-damaging foods and drinks? Take a guess, then read this!

"

DESCRIPTION

Summer is a great opportunity to write a blog. It doesn't have to be long. One or two paragraphs about summer foods that can be damaging to teeth.

LINK: **WWW.RACHELMELE.COM/6-9**

Summer Vacation

SAY THIS

HAPPY SUMMER!

Where are you spending your summer vacation? Comment Below.

"

DESCRIPTION

Encourage followers to post content on your wall! Don't forget to comment back on their posts with personal responses!

LINK: WWW.RACHELMELE.COM/6-10

Video

SAY THIS

Dr. Teeth & the Electric Mayhem!

Love the Muppets!

,,

DESCRIPTION

Feature a funny video your followers and their children will appreciate like the video in this link.

LINK: WWW.RACHELMELE.COM/6-11

Informational Video

SAY THIS

Do you know what's great about fluoride?
Watch this great video from the American
Dental Association to find out.

,,

DESCRIPTION

The American Dental Association is a
wonderful resource for topics.
Subscribe to the "ADA Morning Huddle"
email for daily ideas.

LINK: **WWW.RACHELMELE.COM/6-12**

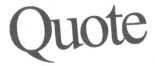

SAY THIS

"You don't have to brush your teeth

- just the ones you want to keep."

~Author Unknown

"

DESCRIPTION

Get creative with this post and ask a
young patient to say it on video or get a
video of your doctor!

LINK: **WWW.RACHELMELE.COM/6-13**

Summer Selfie

SAY THIS

Congrats to [winning family] winners of the Show Us Your Smile Contest! Look at those great smiles! Enjoy your [Prize] from [Practice Name]!

,,

DESCRIPTION

Create a contest for families to participate in. For example, you could have them send their summer vacation photos to be entered to win a prize in any amount or type.

LINK: **WWW.RACHELMELE.COM/6-14**

National Smile Power Day

SAY THIS

Smile Power Day is today! Let's see your big, friendly SMILES posted here on our Facebook page in honor of the day and don't forget to schedule you teeth whitening today!

,,

DESCRIPTION

Encourage followers to post content on your wall! Don't forget to comment back on their posts.

LINK: **WWW.RACHELMELE.COM/6-15**

Spirit Day

SAY THIS

Today is Spirit Day at [Practice Name]!
Help us figure out which team member had
the most spirit! Like your favorite team
member's spirit!

"

DESCRIPTION

Add individual pictures of team members
displaying their spirit and let followers vote
by likes who they like the best!

LINK: WWW.RACHELMELE.COM/6-16

Happy Father's Day

SAY THIS

Share your best happy moments with #Dad and #Win

exciting #Prizes. It can be absolutely anything –

your outings, your secrets, or your pranks together.

#Winners will be announced on Father's Day!   Rules: 1.

Like our page 2. Like & Share this post

3. Hashtag #[PracticeName]DentalCare & #FathersDay

99

DESCRIPTION

Hold a contest to get your followers

involved and promote your practice!

Provide rules, prizes and deadlines in

your social post or on your blog or

website.

LINK: **WWW.RACHELMELE.COM/6-17**

Dental Fun

SAY THIS

This one is a post for all you Elvis fans.
Did you know that Elvis was
obsessed with brushing his teeth? Any of you
obsessed with teeth brushing?

"

DESCRIPTION

Search a picture of Elvis's pearly whites
to add to your fun fact.

LINK: WWW.RACHELMELE.COM/6-18

Active Kids

As a parent, it can be scary when your child falls and hits [his/her] mouth. It is important to have a trusted dentist to call when a dental emergency arises. Call [Practice Name] when a dental emergency arises! Click here for an emergency guide of teeth!

"

DESCRIPTION

Include the phone number to the practice and link to article.

LINK: **WWW.RACHELMELE.COM/6-19**

Dental Fun

SAY THIS

Like tattoos? How would you feel about one on your tooth? Tattoos for teeth are the next body art trend! Would you ever get one? Tag someone that will!

,,

DESCRIPTION

Expose your followers to new and fun trends! Ask them their opinion and encourage them to tag other friends.

LINK: WWW.RACHELMELE.COM/6-20

For Kids

SAY THIS

Teaching your kids to brush their teeth?

Then this is the perfect video for them to watch!

Tag someone who needs this for their kids!

,,

DESCRIPTION

Insert link of video in post! Make
sure you connect with followers if
they leave any comments!

LINK: WWW.RACHELMELE.COM/6-21

Today's Openings

SAY THIS

Hello from [Practice Name].

We have some open appointments at [Time].

Call now to reserve your spot!

Share this post for 10% off your next cleaning!

99

DESCRIPTION

Limit these kinds of posts to only on occasion.

LINK: WWW.RACHELMELE.COM/6-22

Dental

Summer Party

SAY THIS

[Practice Name] knows how to throw a

"Summer Party."

We had a great day of food and

fun with this fantastic team!

,,

DESCRIPTION

Capture photo(s) of team members

enjoying themselves!

LINK: **WWW.RACHELMELE.COM/6-23**

Dentist Beach Day

SAY THIS

This is how dentists do a beach day!

"

DESCRIPTION

Get a picture of the doctors in their bathing suits enjoying a day at the beach. Make it dental related by having them brush their teeth while they are there.

LINK: WWW.RACHELMELE.COM/6-24

Tooth Banking

SAY THIS

Check out this news about the gaining acceptance of tooth banking. Would you do this?

"

DESCRIPTION

Keep your followers up to date with the latest trends. Include a link to this article or others about tooth banking.

LINK: **WWW.RACHELMELE.COM/6-25**

Summer Dance Video

---- SAY THIS ----

Summer break is getting the best of us!

What happens after hours at [Practice Name]?

Sometimes we just have to

end the day with a dance off.

,,

---- DESCRIPTION ----

Record a video of your team members
having fun in a dance off session, check
the video below for ideas.

LINK: **WWW.RACHELMELE.COM/6-26**

Dental College Tips

SAY THIS

Hey Parents! Read about these

Dental Care Tips for College Bound Teens!

Make sure to schedule your teen's appointment

(or remind them to) before they are off at

college eating whatever they want!

,,

DESCRIPTION

Write your own dental blog post featuring
the tips and tricks of maintaining great
oral health while being away at college!
Encourage your followers to tag their
teens so they can read about it, too!

LINK: **WWW.RACHELMELE.COM/6-27**

Insurance Awareness Day

SAY THIS

It's Insurance Awareness Day:

[Practice Name] accepts many insurance programs.

Call us with any of your insurance questions!

,,

DESCRIPTION

Provide your followers with a list of all the insurance programs your practice accepts. This is a good way to expose the practice to future patients.

LINK: WWW.RACHELMELE.COM/6-28

Quote

SAY THIS

"People seldom notice old clothes if you wear a big smile." ~Lee Mildon

,,

DESCRIPTION

Consider creating a unique graphic with the quote on it instead of just posting the words alone. Or ask someone to take a video explaining why the quote is important to them.

LINK: WWW.RACHELMELE.COM/6-29

Social Media Day

SAY THIS

Happy Social Media Day to all of our friends and fans! We love that social media has given us another way to stay in touch with you! Thanks for connecting with us!

"

DESCRIPTION

Social Media plays a big part in every industry, thank all your followers for their loyalty both online and in the office.

LINK: **WWW.RACHELMELE.COM/6-30**

Question

SAY THIS

50% of people say that a smile is the first feature they notice about someone! Any thoughts on what the other 50% notice first?

,,

DESCRIPTION

Have your followers respond and answer the question. At the end of the day post the results of your survey. Include a photo of someone smiling from ear to ear in your post.

LINK: **WWW.RACHELMELE.COM/7-1**

Dental Fun

SAY THIS

38.5 = the total days an average American

spends brushing teeth over a lifetime.

[Practice Name] recommends brushing

At least 2x a day and immediately after meals.

"

DESCRIPTION

Upload a video or photo of a flipping

calendar to highlight the point.

LINK: **WWW.RACHELMELE.COM/7-2**

4th of July Video

SAY THIS

Here's an Independence Day music video from our office. Happy Independence Day, and don't forget to floss.

,,

DESCRIPTION

Take a short video of the office staff singing this Independence Day song. Add your own dental twist to it.

LINK: **WWW.RACHELMELE.COM/7-3**

4th of July

SAY THIS

Happy Independence Day.

Did you know George Washington's dentures were not made of wood as commonly believed?

"

DESCRIPTION

Include a photo of a team member pointing to a picture of George Washington.

LINK: WWW.RACHELMELE.COM/7-4

Question

SAY THIS

With all the talk on the news about Zika,

we wondered– do you know

how many teeth a mosquito has?

What's your best guess?

"

DESCRIPTION

Answer: 47 teeth.

Add a photo of a mosquito smiling.

LINK: WWW.RACHELMELE.COM/7-5

Contest

SAY THIS

To celebrate the summer,

we're giving away a dental monogrammed

tumbler. For your chance to win, tell us your

favorite summer beverage.

99

DESCRIPTION

Include a link to this or a similar

dental monogrammed tumbler.

LINK: **WWW.RACHELMELE.COM/7-6**

Question

SAY THIS

We have a summer teeth quiz for you

from the American Dental Association.

Take the quiz and post below

how many you got correct.

"

DESCRIPTION

Use this quiz from the American Dental Association or come up with your own quiz.

LINK: **WWW.RACHELMELE.COM/7-7**

No Cavity Club

SAY THIS

Congrats to [Patient Name] who joins the No Cavity Club list. Time for a prize.

99

DESCRIPTION

Congratulate your patients (young and old) for being part of your No Cavity Club.

LINK: WWW.RACHELMELE.COM/7-8

Dental Fun

SAY THIS

This is too funny. Crest® fans rocked the @AARP convention with a Flash Mob!

"

DESCRIPTION

Check out the video and then share it with your patients on social media.

LINK: **WWW.RACHELMELE.COM/7-9**

Running Late

SAY THIS

Running late for your dental appointment? Just give us a call. We don't want you to have to pull a Mr. Bean.

,,

DESCRIPTION

This video of Mr. Bean getting dressed goes perfectly with a social message reminding patients to just call if they are running late.

LINK: **WWW.RACHELMELE.COM/7-10**

Doctor Fun

SAY THIS

[Doctor(s) Name(s)] went for a

hike today and left a trail.

--- 99 ---

DESCRIPTION

Grab some tooth brushes and put them on a

hiking trail, take a picture and include it with

this post.

LINK: WWW.RACHELMELE.COM/7-11

Pop Quiz

SAY THIS

Pop Quiz! In the movie "The Great Gatsby," which character has cufflinks made of molars?

,,

DESCRIPTION

Answer: Meyer Wolfsheim, one of Gatsby's underworld connections. Molar cuff links are for sale. Link to pictures.

LINK: **WWW.RACHELMELE.COM/7-12**

Embrace Your Geekiness Day

SAY THIS

Embrace Your Geekiness Day! What's your favorite geeky toy?

,,

DESCRIPTION

Stage a photo of a staff member wearing geeky classes holding their iPhone or another gadget or purchase a geeky photo online.

LINK: **WWW.RACHELMELE.COM/7-13**

Refer a Friend

SAY THIS

[Practice Name] thanks our patients who refer their friends with a [Prize].

Thanks for telling your friends and family about our practice.

"

DESCRIPTION

Grab kid's blocks, spell "Refer a Friend" and then take a picture to include with this post or purchase a photo online.

LINK: **WWW.RACHELMELE.COM/7-14**

Contest

SAY THIS

[Practice Name] is giving away this water bottle. Comment below on how much water you drink a day for your chance to win.

,,

DESCRIPTION

Link to this or another

dental themed water bottle.

LINK: **WWW.RACHELMELE.COM/7-15**

Dental Fun

SAY THIS

Did you know, toothbrush bristles were originally made from animal hairs?

"

DESCRIPTION

If you live in an area with cows, get your camera out.   Or purchase this super cute cow photo online.

LINK: WWW.RACHELMELE.COM/7-16

Summer Fun

SAY THIS

Summer is here and that means it's time for summer vacation. Anyone have plans to visit the world's largest tooth in Trenton, NJ this summer? If you are close by, be sure to tag us!

"

DESCRIPTION

Include an image of the world's largest tooth. Even better, get a picture with the doctor or a team member visiting this tooth.

LINK: **WWW.RACHELMELE.COM/7-17**

Dental Fun

SAY THIS

It's getting hot out there.

Anyone want a dip in this tooth shaped pool?

"

DESCRIPTION

Include a link in your post to a

tooth shaped pool.

LINK: **WWW.RACHELMELE.COM/7-18**

Question

SAY THIS

Floss picks or traditional floss?

Tell us which is your favorite?

,,

DESCRIPTION

Grab a floss pick and traditional floss, put them on a piece of paper with the word "OR" in-between. Take a picture and include it with this post.

LINK: WWW.RACHELMELE.COM/7-19

Summer Contest

SAY THIS

Summer Scavenger Hunt. Come into the office to get a list of activities visiting local businesses to win $100.

"

DESCRIPTION

Send your patients to local businesses and have them take a picture there, post it on social and tag your practice. This is a great way to get the community to support your practice. Alert the businesses in advance to approve contest participation.

LINK: **WWW.RACHELMELE.COM/7-20**

Junk Food Day

SAY THIS

Today is National Junk Food Day!

Don't forget to brush and floss your teeth.

Don't forget to wash away the JUNK FOOD

that might get stuck between your teeth!

"

DESCRIPTION

Get a team member to eat some junk food, getting it all over her face.   With a guilty look on her face, take a photo and post it here.   Or, take a photo of a table full of junk food.

LINK: **WWW.RACHELMELE.COM/7-21**

Oral Cancer Awareness

SAY THIS

The average dentist will save the life of 11 patients in their life by identifying a potential risk of oral cancer. Our office takes an extra two minutes to screen all our patients for oral cancer.

"

DESCRIPTION

Patients want to know that you will take care of them. Sharing with your patients that you are looking out for their well being goes a long way.

LINK: **WWW.RACHELMELE.COM/7-22**

Fluoride

SAY THIS

Got questions about fluoride for your children? We have answers.

99

DESCRIPTION

The ADA has a great article about fluoride for children. This may be a good topic for a blog also.

LINK: **WWW.RACHELMELE.COM/7-23**

Contest

SAY THIS

Who do you know who wears the "best" socks? Tag them here to enter them to win a pair of teeth socks. The most likes wins.

,,

DESCRIPTION

Include a photo of team members with fun socks. Track tags and respond, and then post the winner by counting likes.

LINK: **WWW.RACHELMELE.COM/7-24**

Invisalign Teen®

SAY THIS

Justin Bieber circa 2011 getting

Invisalign Teen ®

,,

DESCRIPTION

Include a link to this video of Justin Bieber

showing off his Invisalign Teen® aligners.

LINK: **WWW.RACHELMELE.COM/7-25**

Dental Fun

SAY THIS

It's Mick Jagger's birthday.

Mick Jagger has a diamond

implanted in his tooth.

"

DESCRIPTION

This video shows Mick Jagger talking about his diamond implanted tooth. Link to it.

LINK: WWW.RACHELMELE.COM/7-26

White Teeth

SAY THIS

Who wants white teeth?

Here's our report on the benefits of

apple cider vinegar for teeth whitening.

,,

DESCRIPTION

Create your own video talking about the

benefits of apple cider vinegar or link to

this one.

LINK: **WWW.RACHELMELE.COM/7-27**

Brush After Lunch

SAY THIS

Click "Like" if you brush your teeth after lunch!

,,

DESCRIPTION

Take a picture of the whole team brushing their teeth at the same time or purchase this photo.

LINK: WWW.RACHELMELE.COM/7-28

Toothbrush Song

SAY THIS

It's not every day a toothbrush gets featured in a Top 40 song. Just goes to show how important toothbrushes are. Check out this video from DNCE with their song, "Toothbrush."

"

DESCRIPTION

Watch the video and include a link in your post.

LINK: **WWW.RACHELMELE.COM/7-29**

Dental Fun

SAY THIS

Are you great at chess?

How about a game of chess on this

dental chess board?

,,

DESCRIPTION

Link to an example of a

chess board made for dentistry.

LINK: WWW.RACHELMELE.COM/7-30

Celebrities

SAY THIS

Check out these celebrity

before and after tooth transformations.

Who do you think has the best smile?

"

DESCRIPTION

Search the Internet for your favorite celebrity before and after photos or include this link in your post. Respond to all replies.

LINK: WWW.RACHELMELE.COM/7-31

Question

SAY THIS

Do you have a mysterious toothbrush

in the bathroom that no one in your family uses?

Post a picture of it here.

,,

DESCRIPTION

Post a picture of a lonely toothbrush not in
the toothbrush holder.

LINK: WWW.RACHELMELE.COM/8-1

Dental Heels

SAY THIS

Ladies, need a new pair of heels? How about these teeth shoes?

""

DESCRIPTION

Link to a picture of these
super crazy high heel shoes made of teeth.

LINK: **WWW.RACHELMELE.COM/8-2**

Giving Back

SAY THIS

Our practice supports the American Academy of Cosmetic Dentistry Charitable Foundation. Give back a smile.

,,

DESCRIPTION

Any time your practice contributes to a cause, be sure to let your patients know.

LINK: WWW.RACHELMELE.COM/8-3

Tooth Fairy

SAY THIS

Check out this absolutely adorable video with the tooth fairy.

"

DESCRIPTION

Include a link to YouTube sharing this tooth fairy video or create your own video.

LINK: WWW.RACHELMELE.COM/8-4

Dental Chairs

SAY THIS

We are thinking about getting some

new dental chairs for our office.

What do you think of this one?

,,

DESCRIPTION

Find a super old photo of a dental office chair

(circa 1915) and include it with your post.

LINK: WWW.RACHELMELE.COM/8-5

Question

SAY THIS

Pop Quiz!

What causes cavities?

Click on this link to get a fun explanation.

"

DESCRIPTION

Get [Practice Doctor(s)] to hold a sign saying

"What Causes Cavities,"

take a picture for sharing and

add a link to the video.

LINK: **WWW.RACHELMELE.COM/8-6**

Chewing Celery

SAY THIS

Did you know chewing celery helps in producing more saliva in your mouth which prevents plaque? Eating celery once a week can help keep your teeth naturally clean on top of brushing. Guess who loves celery in our practice?

"

DESCRIPTION

Post a picture of a staff member chewing celery.

LINK: **WWW.RACHELMELE.COM/8-7**

Soda Teeth

SAY THIS

What do you think happens when you put teeth in soda? Click here to find out.

,,

DESCRIPTION

Link this video or do your own experiment on video and share it.

LINK: **WWW.RACHELMELE.COM/8-8**

Kids Oral Health

SAY THIS

Here are some fun coloring pages from

the American Dental Association

to help kids with good oral health.

,,

DESCRIPTION

Share these in the office or have your followers

print them out for their children.

LINK: WWW.RACHELMELE.COM/8-9

Justin Bieber Video

SAY THIS

Check out our practice singing our version of a Justin Bieber song, "Braces, Braces, Braces, No"

,,

DESCRIPTION

Take a video of your practice singing Justin Bieber's song "Baby," but with your own lyrics about braces and Invisalign.

LINK: WWW.RACHELMELE.COM/8-10

Kids Toothpaste

SAY THIS

These toothpastes may be perfect for your little one.

Check them out.

,,

DESCRIPTION

Link to the toothpaste products you

recommend for your little patients.

LINK: **WWW.RACHELMELE.COM/8-11**

Lemons!

SAY THIS

Do you love lemons?

[Practice Name] explains why you

might want to rethink liking them.

,,

DESCRIPTION

Get practice doctors or another team

member to explain in a video why lemons

can be harmful to your teeth.

LINK: **WWW.RACHELMELE.COM/8-12**

True or False

SAY THIS

True or False:

You can have gingivitis in some areas

of your mouth and not others.

,,

DESCRIPTION

Take a photo or video of practice doctors

asking this question.

LINK: **WWW.RACHELMELE.COM/8-13**

Throw Back Thursday

SAY THIS

#TBT to some of the best of the best in dental cartoon education.

99

DESCRIPTION

Watch and post a video of these dental themed cartoons.

LINK: **WWW.RACHELMELE.COM/8-14**

Video

SAY THIS

We caught [Practice Doctor] attempting to rap.

"

DESCRIPTION

Dentists can have fun too.

Create your own version of any popular song.

LINK: **WWW.RACHELMELE.COM/8-15**

Tell a Joke Day

SAY THIS

It's National Tell a Joke Day. Here's [Practice Team Member] with one of our favorites.

What game do you play if you don't take care of your teeth? Answer: Tooth or Consequences!

"

DESCRIPTION

Take a video of a team member telling this joke. Embed the text of the joke in the video as well to accommodate for patients who don't like to turn their volume up.

LINK: WWW.RACHELMELE.COM/8-16

Dental Movie Scene

SAY THIS

What's your favorite TV or Movie Dental scene?

,,

DESCRIPTION

Include a link to this scene from

"Finding Nemo."

LINK: **WWW.RACHELMELE.COM/8-17**

Patient Review

SAY THIS

We love that our patients love us.
Check out what [Patient Name] had to say about us:

99

DESCRIPTION

Ask a patient to do a testimonial video

for your practice.

LINK: **WWW.RACHELMELE.COM/8-18**

Back to School

SAY THIS

[Practice Doctor(s)] want to answer your questions regarding your child's back to school dental visit.

"

DESCRIPTION

Create your list to inform followers and possibly add this to a blog.

LINK: **WWW.RACHELMELE.COM/8-19**

Toothbrush Holder

SAY THIS

Where does your toothbrush live?

It could live in this Tooth Shaped Holder.

Tell us below why your toothbrush deserves to

win this holder.

,,

DESCRIPTION

Include a link to a tooth shaped toothbrush
holder like this one.

LINK: **WWW.RACHELMELE.COM/8-20**

Dental Recipes

SAY THIS

Having a healthy diet can have an impact on your oral health. It's not JUST about brushing your teeth twice a day. Here is a healthy recipe from the Food Network®.

99

DESCRIPTION

Share any of your favorite receipts with your patients. If you have a practice cook book, be sure to share that too.

LINK: **WWW.RACHELMELE.COM/8-21**

Yearbook Fun

SAY THIS

Any guesses who this awkward kid is?

Post your awkward yearbook photos below.

"

DESCRIPTION

Post a picture of the doctors yearbook photo or create a collage of everyone and ask your patients to guess who is who.

LINK: **WWW.RACHELMELE.COM/8-22**

Team Congratulations

SAY THIS

[Practice Team Member Name] just had a baby girl.

Congrats to on the birth of [Newborn Name].

We hope [he/she] loves [his/her] new [gift].

99

DESCRIPTION

Send [team member name] this tooth

blanket or something like it and post a

picture of baby with their new gift.

LINK: **WWW.RACHELMELE.COM/8-23**

Dental Implants

SAY THIS

Here is some interesting information

regarding dental implants.

Call us at [Practice Phone #]

if you have any questions.

,,

DESCRIPTION

Keep your followers informed and

consider this topic for a blog.

LINK: **WWW.RACHELMELE.COM/8-24**

First Dental Exam

SAY THIS

According to the American Academy of Pediatric Dentistry, children should have a dental exam by their first birthday. Here's our newest patient.

"

DESCRIPTION

Post a picture (with the parent's written permission) of your youngest patient.

LINK: **WWW.RACHELMELE.COM/8-25**

National Dog Day

SAY THIS

In honor of National Dog Day,

we want to see pictures

of you brushing your pooch's teeth.

"

DESCRIPTION

Get a team member to take a photo of their

dog getting his teeth brushed.

LINK: **WWW.RACHELMELE.COM/8-26**

Patient Spotlight

SAY THIS

[Patient Name] has been

a patient of ours since [Date].

Thanks [Patient Name] for

letting us take care of your oral health.

"

DESCRIPTION

Post a picture of Doctor and Patient.

LINK: WWW.RACHELMELE.COM/8-27

Question

SAY THIS

Do you still use an "old school" toothbrush?

"

DESCRIPTION

Post a video of your practice showing off
the practice's recommended electric
toothbrush or link to this video.

LINK: **WWW.RACHELMELE.COM/8-28**

Football Season

SAY THIS

In preparation for football season,

[Practice Doctor(s)] visited the

[Local School] to fit the

student athletes with mouth guards.

,,

DESCRIPTION

Take a photo or video of [Practice Doctor(s)]

giving student athletes their mouth guards.

Similar to this video.

LINK: WWW.RACHELMELE.COM/8-29

Charitable Giving

SAY THIS

Our wonderful team has decided to support this great [cause]. Come out and support us.

"

DESCRIPTION

Take a photo of the practice doctor(s) and team practicing for a charity run.

LINK: **WWW.RACHELMELE.COM/8-30**

Toothbrush

SAY THIS

*Our practice recommends the Sonicare
AirFloss® to remove plaque between your teeth.
Call our office if you don't have yours yet.
[Practice Phone #]*

,,

DESCRIPTION

Take a photo or video of someone from your
office using this or another recommended
product.

LINK: **WWW.RACHELMELE.COM/8-31**

Dental Fun

SAY THIS

When choosing your dentist, we highly recommend not choosing this one...

,,

DESCRIPTION

This video from Dean Martin, Ken Lane and Foster Brooks is a classic. Patients will get a kick out of it.

LINK: **WWW.RACHELMELE.COM/9-1**

Bacon Day

SAY THIS

Ever tried bacon flavored toothpaste?

#IntlBaconDay

99

DESCRIPTION

Purchase a tube of bacon flavored toothpaste
and get one person or the whole office to
react to it on video.

LINK: WWW.RACHELMELE.COM/9-2

Toothbrush

SAY THIS

Which is best? Hard or soft toothbrushes? [Practice Doctor] explains.

,,

DESCRIPTION

Take a short 30-60 second video of [Practice Doctor] explaining why soft bristle toothbrushes are the best.

LINK: WWW.RACHELMELE.COM/9-3

Self-Improvement Month

SAY THIS

September is Self-Improvement Month. [Practice Doctor(s)] set a goal of reading two new books a month for a full year. What are your self-improvement goals?

99

DESCRIPTION

Take a picture of [Practice Doctor(s)] in action working on self-improvement or download this link.

LINK: **WWW.RACHELMELE.COM/9-4**

Back to School

SAY THIS

It's back to school time. Be sure to get your mouth guard to protect your teeth from injury during this year's sports season.

,,

DESCRIPTION

Ask a patient who is an athlete to take a photo wearing his/her mouth guard holding a prop like a football or soccer ball.

LINK: WWW.RACHELMELE.COM/9-5

Procrastination Day

SAY THIS

In honor of National Procrastination Day, we'd like to remind you to call and schedule your appointment today. [Practice Phone Number]

,,

DESCRIPTION

Take a picture of a staff member with their feet up on the desk (on a stack of papers) and hands behind their head.

LINK: WWW.RACHELMELE.COM/9-6

National Gum Care Month

SAY THIS

September is National Gum Care Month. Call our office to schedule an appointment and take care of those gums! [Practice Phone Number]

99

DESCRIPTION

Stitch together separate photos of each team member pointing at their gums.

LINK: **WWW.RACHELMELE.COM/9-7**

Dental Fun

SAY THIS

Our office had a dance

party today.

99

DESCRIPTION

Get creative and create a fun video like this
one of your practice dancing and having fun.

LINK: **WWW.RACHELMELE.COM/9-8**

Heart Health

SAY THIS

[Practice Doctor(s)] on dental and heart health.

"

DESCRIPTION

Read the linked article below and then blog about in your own words or create a video or simply share this link.

LINK: **WWW.RACHELMELE.COM/9-9**

Practice Promotion

SAY THIS

You are never too old to have a beautiful smile and we can help. Call our office at [Practice Phone Number]

"

DESCRIPTION

Purchase a stock photo of an adult smiling or ask a patient if you can take a photo of them for this social message.

LINK: WWW.RACHELMELE.COM/9-10

Contest

SAY THIS

We are giving away a monogrammed tooth koozie. Just comment below with the first word that pops into your head when you think of [Practice Name].

"

DESCRIPTION

Purchase these great koozies at any promotional shop.

LINK: **WWW.RACHELMELE.COM/9-11**

Dental Fun

SAY THIS

Even superheroes brush their teeth.
This video proves it.

,,

DESCRIPTION

This video of a playdough version of the
Hulk and Elsa from "Frozen" illustrates
why it's so important to brush.

LINK: **WWW.RACHELMELE.COM/9-12**

Team Appreciation

SAY THIS

[Practice Team Member]'s title is Dental Office Manager only because full-time multitasking ninja is not an actual job title.

"

DESCRIPTION

Purchase this shirt for your office manager and post a picture of her wearing it.

LINK: **WWW.RACHELMELE.COM/9-13**

Brushing App

SAY THIS

Do you brush and floss twice a day? Maybe you need the Brush DJ app which plays 2 minutes of your favorite song. Check it out.

99

DESCRIPTION

Link straight to the video or create your own video showing how you use the app.

LINK: **WWW.RACHELMELE.COM/9-14**

Dental Fun

SAY THIS

Get rid of your dental nasties.

99

DESCRIPTION

Colgate created a great video with youngsters explaining how to get rid of "nasties."

LINK: WWW.RACHELMELE.COM/9-15

Dental Game

SAY THIS

Ever tried the mouth guard

challenge?

,,

DESCRIPTION

This is fun for everyone. Get your

patients involved.

LINK: **WWW.RACHELMELE.COM/9-16**

Blog

SAY THIS

Do you know what a geographic tongue is?
Check out our latest blog to learn more.

99

DESCRIPTION

This topic is great for a blog.

LINK: WWW.RACHELMELE.COM/9-17

Cavity

SAY THIS

78% of Americans have had at least 1 cavity by age 17. Dare to share how many you have had?

"

DESCRIPTION

Here are some images to help make your point. Respond to your followers' replies.

LINK: WWW.RACHELMELE.COM/9-18

Dental Fun

SAY THIS

What makes you SMILE?

"

DESCRIPTION

Put those words on a smile with a team member holding it and have the answer for each team member.

LINK: WWW.RACHELMELE.COM/9-19

Love Your Teeth Day

SAY THIS

Happy Love Your Teeth Day! XOXO, no one loves your teeth more than we do!

,,

DESCRIPTION

Download a 'love your teeth' image from istockphoto, or any stock image site. Or take your own photo.

LINK: **WWW.RACHELMELE.COM/9-20**

Local Business Promotion

SAY THIS

We absolutely love [Local Coffee Shop]. Thanks for making the best latte around.

"

DESCRIPTION

Post a photo of staff at your local coffee shop or business. Be sure to tag the business at the same time. They may tag you back.

LINK: **WWW.RACHELMELE.COM/9-21**

Toothbrush

SAY THIS

Treat your toothbrush like your password!

,,

DESCRIPTION

Take a picture of a staff member not sharing their toothbrush.

LINK: WWW.RACHELMELE.COM/9-22

Local School Visit

SAY THIS

[Practice Name] is headed to [Local School] today to teach the 2nd graders how to properly brush and floss their teeth.

,,

DESCRIPTION

Take a video of practice doctors at the school or at least some awesome group shots.

LINK: WWW.RACHELMELE.COM/9-23

1st Day of Fall

SAY THIS

Tomorrow is the first official day of Fall!
What about this season makes you smile?

99

DESCRIPTION

Share important fall calendar dates.

LINK: WWW.RACHELMELE.COM/9-24

Dental Facts

SAY THIS

Why do we lose teeth? Check out this information.

,,

DESCRIPTION

Give your patients some interesting facts.

Make it unique to your practice.

LINK: WWW.RACHELMELE.COM/9-25

Smile Exercise

SAY THIS

Have you been doing your smiling exercises?
Your emotions may be tied to your smile.

,,

DESCRIPTION

Include a picture of the team doing their
smiling exercises or create your own video.

LINK: WWW.RACHELMELE.COM/9-26

Braces

SAY THIS

Do you know how braces work? Watch

this video to see.

„

DESCRIPTION

Share interesting, instructional

information with your followers.

LINK: **WWW.RACHELMELE.COM/9-27**

Good Neighbor Day

SAY THIS

Today is National Good Neighbor Day! Be a good neighbor today, all you have to do is SMILE! :D

,,

DESCRIPTION

Who is your practice neighbor? Stop by with something sweet and document the moment on social.

LINK: **WWW.RACHELMELE.COM/9-28**

National Coffee Day

SAY THIS

Today is National Coffee Day! We've added some fun flavors at our coffee bar. Check them out.

99

DESCRIPTION

If you have a coffee area in your practice, show it off on National Coffee Day.

LINK: **WWW.RACHELMELE.COM/9-29**

Apple a Day

SAY THIS

An apple a day won't keep the dentist away. Did you know apples can be as bad for your teeth as sweets and fizzy drinks?

,,

DESCRIPTION

Tell the story of how apples can be harmful for teeth in a quick 30 second video or link to this article.

LINK: WWW.RACHELMELE.COM/9-30

Dental Hygiene Month

SAY THIS

October is Dental Hygiene
Month. Don't you just love
our hygienists?

"

DESCRIPTION

Post a group photo of hygienists doing
something fun.

LINK: **WWW.RACHELMELE.COM/10-1**

Breast Cancer Awareness

--- SAY THIS ---

Everyone is wearing PINK, PINK, PINK today in honor of breast cancer awareness.

"

--- DESCRIPTION ---

Get the whole team dressed in pink for a group shot.

LINK: WWW.RACHELMELE.COM/10-2

Halloween

SAY THIS

It's almost time for Halloween. Do you have your costume picked out yet? Here's an easy way to make a toothpaste costume.

99

DESCRIPTION

Include a link to this video with instructions or create your own video.

LINK: **WWW.RACHELMELE.COM/10-3**

Toothbrush

SAY THIS

The seasons are changing. Now is a good time to change your toothbrush. We recommend every 3 months. How often do you change your toothbrush?

99

DESCRIPTION

You might have followers come into your office to pick up a new toothbrush.

LINK: **WWW.RACHELMELE.COM/10-4**

Dental Fun

SAY THIS

*We had one of our patients ask us today,
"can you pause the movie until I come
back next time?"*

99

DESCRIPTION

Take a photo of a patient watching a
movie or the TV.

LINK: WWW.RACHELMELE.COM/10-5

World Smile Day

SAY THIS

It's WORLD SMILE DAY! For every smile posted below, we'll donate $1 to [Cause].

#WorldSmileDay

,,

DESCRIPTION

Take and post a picture that supports your cause.

LINK: WWW.RACHELMELE.COM/10-6

National X-Ray Day

SAY THIS

It's National X-Ray Day. Here's why dental x-rays are an important tool in detecting damage and disease.

"

DESCRIPTION

Show off your x-ray machine in a picture or show [Practice Doctor(s)] sharing an x-ray with a patient.

LINK: WWW.RACHELMELE.COM/10-7

Cold & Flu

SAY THIS

Fall is here and with it comes the dreaded cold and flu season. After recovering from your cold, we will tell you one of the most important steps you can take to avoid becoming re-infected is replacing your toothbrush!

,,

DESCRIPTION

Consider getting flu shots for the team and posting a picture.

LINK: WWW.RACHELMELE.COM/10-8

Tooth Fairy

SAY THIS

We want to know how you spend your tooth fairy money. Post below via message or video. Here's what these kiddos do:

"

DESCRIPTION

This adorable video will put a smile on anyone's face.

LINK: WWW.RACHELMELE.COM/10-9

Columbus Day

SAY THIS

Come by the office and share our salute

to Columbus Day.

"

DESCRIPTION

Link to a picture of these

little "ships."

LINK: WWW.RACHELMELE.COM/10-10

Contest

SAY THIS

Patients, please decorate small pumpkins to be entered into a Facebook contest. Voting takes place on Facebook through comments. Each pumpkin is numbered. Facebook friends comment on photos with their vote.

,,

DESCRIPTION

This is also a fun way to decorate your office for October. Click through the photos on the link to see ideas.

LINK: **WWW.RACHELMELE.COM/10-11**

Toothbrush Sharing

SAY THIS

While we don't recommend sharing your toothbrush, this is pretty darn cute.

99

DESCRIPTION

These two twins argue over who gets to use the toothbrush. Who can resist!

LINK: **WWW.RACHELMELE.COM/10-12**

Country Western Day

SAY THIS

It's Country Western Day at [Practice Name]. Be sure to wear your country gear if you have an appointment today.

,,

DESCRIPTION

Display a picture of the team in Country Western garb or a fun "Western" photo.

LINK: **WWW.RACHELMELE.COM/10-13**

Dental Nails

SAY THIS

[Practice Team Member], our receptionist got her nails done with a dental theme.

"

DESCRIPTION

Have a team member get their nails done with a dental theme like the nails in the link below, take a picture and post it.

LINK: WWW.RACHELMELE.COM/10-14

Boss's Day

SAY THIS

For Boss's Day, the team at [Practice Name] wants to say a very big thank you to the best boss in the world, [Practice Doctor(s)]! Thank you!

,,

DESCRIPTION

This practice got each team member to say happy boss's day in a short, simple video.

LINK: **WWW.RACHELMELE.COM/10-15**

Root Canal

SAY THIS

What does root canal treatment entail?

,,

DESCRIPTION

Help your followers understand the benefits of dentistry.

LINK: **WWW.RACHELMELE.COM/10-16**

Flossing

SAY THIS

Should you floss before or after you brush your teeth??

"

DESCRIPTION

Create a sign that says "before or after" with a team member tilting their head in wonder.

LINK: **WWW.RACHELMELE.COM/10-17**

Sugar-free Gum

SAY THIS

What's your favorite sugar-free gum?
Here's [Practice Team Member]
explaining why the [Practice Name]
team chews sugar-free.

"

DESCRIPTION

Create a short 30-60 second
video explaining the benefits of
sugar-free gum.

LINK: **WWW.RACHELMELE.COM/10-18**

Office View

SAY THIS

The trees outside our office are in full bloom. Share scenes of beauty you see around the area with all of us.

,,

DESCRIPTION

Post your practice with the fall foliage in the background.

LINK: **WWW.RACHELMELE.COM/10-19**

Sugary Soda

SAY THIS

True or false: People who drink 3 or more sugary sodas daily have 62% more dental decay, fillings, and tooth loss. "Sip all day, get decay!"

""

DESCRIPTION

Take a video of multiple team members getting caught red handed drinking soda.

LINK: **WWW.RACHELMELE.COM/10-20**

Team Recognition

SAY THIS

We want to congratulate our [Practice Team Member], who completed [his/her] first 1/2 marathon.

--- 🙶 ---

DESCRIPTION

Post a picture of team member completing the race.

LINK: **WWW.RACHELMELE.COM/10-21**

Dental Implants

SAY THIS

Do you know the advantages of dental implants?.

"

DESCRIPTION

Let your followers know the kinds of procedures available in your office.

LINK: **WWW.RACHELMELE.COM/10-22**

Patient Before & After

SAY THIS

We couldn't help posting this before and after of our patient, [Patient Name]. Congrats, [Patient Name] your smile is AMAZING.

,,

DESCRIPTION

Be sure to get written approval before posting. Tag the patient, too.

LINK: WWW.RACHELMELE.COM/10-23

Patient Recognition

SAY THIS

Our patients are incredibly talented. Check out this video of [Patient Name] performing.

"

DESCRIPTION

Anytime you can boast about your exceptional patients, do it. Just be sure you have permission first.

LINK: **WWW.RACHELMELE.COM/10-24**

Team Recognition

SAY THIS

Today, [Practice Team Member], one of our dental assistants is celebrating [# of years] years with our practice. Thank you for helping to make our practice great, [Practice Team Member]!

,,

DESCRIPTION

Recognize and celebrate your team.

LINK: **WWW.RACHELMELE.COM/10-25**

Dental Floss

Did you floss your teeth today? Here are some other ways to use dental floss.

"

DESCRIPTION

Get [Practice Doctor(s)] or a team member to hold up a sign that says, "Did you floss your teeth today" or have them hold floss in their hands.

LINK: WWW.RACHELMELE.COM/10-26

Contest

SAY THIS

Guess the Smile. Can you guess which smile belongs to which team member at our office?

,,

DESCRIPTION

Put all the smiles in one image numbered. Make this a Facebook post. Don't forget to explain the prize and display winners later.

LINK: WWW.RACHELMELE.COM/10-27

National Cat Day

SAY THIS

In honor of National Cat Day, here's a picture of [Practice Team Member]'s cat. Did you know that cats can get dental disease? #CatDay

"

DESCRIPTION

Post a picture of practice doctor's or a team member's cute cat and/or link to this website page.

LINK: **WWW.RACHELMELE.COM/10-28**

Question

Halloween Fun

SAY THIS

How are you dressing for Halloween tomorrow? Here are some Halloween activities.

"

DESCRIPTION

Post a photo of the office team all dressed up for Halloween. This link includes pumpkin carving stencils and activity sheets.

LINK: WWW.RACHELMELE.COM/10-29

Halloween Buy Back

SAY THIS

It's Halloween. [Practice Name] wants to buy your candy! Our goal is to collect 300 pounds. We'll be accepting candy all week long. $1 per pound of unopened candy. We'll be sending all candy to our service members overseas.

"

DESCRIPTION

Pile that candy up on your reception desk for a fun photo.

LINK: **WWW.RACHELMELE.COM/10-30**

Halloween

SAY THIS

We like to share in the Halloween fun. Check
out how the team dressed up this year.

99

DESCRIPTION

Have fun and share the fun with
your patients.

LINK: **WWW.RACHELMELE.COM/10-31**

Aligners

SAY THIS

Smoking is discouraged while wearing aligners because it is possible for the aligners to become discolored.

,,

DESCRIPTION

This photo is a dramatic way to get the point across that smoking can ruin your smile.

LINK: WWW.RACHELMELE.COM/11-1

Movember

SAY THIS

To help kick off Movember, [Practice Doctor(s)] will donate $1 to the American Cancer Society for every patient who posts their growing mustache photo and tags our practice.

"

DESCRIPTION

Wear "mustaches" in the office.

LINK: **WWW.RACHELMELE.COM/11-2**

Daylight Savings

SAY THIS

Daylight saving is ending. Did you know the additional amount of daylight provides vitamin D, also known as the "sunshine vitamin," that could extend the life and health of your teeth and bones?

,,

DESCRIPTION

Link to these tips for daylight saving time.

LINK: WWW.RACHELMELE.COM/11-3

Dental Fun

SAY THIS

Don't be an anti-dentite. [Practice Doctor(s)] is not "just a dentist."

99

DESCRIPTION

Seinfeld episode where Kramer calls Jerry an anti-dentite. So funny.

LINK: WWW.RACHELMELE.COM/11-4

Election Day

SAY THIS

Don't forget to vote! On Tuesday, Nov. 2, 1920, millions of women voted in the elections after the 19th amendment was passed on Aug. 26, 1920, guaranteeing a woman's right to vote, according to History.com.

,,

DESCRIPTION

Zoom in on [Practice Doctor(s)] voting or wearing his/her iVoted sticker.

LINK: **WWW.RACHELMELE.COM/11-5**

Election Day

SAY THIS

With Election Day just around the corner, we decided to ask our youngest patients to explain what Election Day is all about.

"

DESCRIPTION

Take a video asking your young patients to explain Election Day. For more election day post ideas, visit this link.

LINK: **WWW.RACHELMELE.COM/11-6**

Dental Fun

SAY THIS

Guess what toy inspired [Practice Doctor(s)]

to be a dentist?

"

DESCRIPTION

Encourage your patients to pursue

dentistry.

LINK: WWW.RACHELMELE.COM/11-7

Cold Season

SAY THIS

Cold seasons is upon us. Here are some tips from the ADA on how to care for your mouth when you are sick.

99

DESCRIPTION

Let your patients know about your sterilization process in the office.

LINK: **WWW.RACHELMELE.COM/11-8**

Snow Day

SAY THIS

Show us the fun you are having in the snow.

,,

DESCRIPTION

This post describes some fun dental games for snow days. Or create your own. Maybe the team wants to play?

LINK: **WWW.RACHELMELE.COM/11-9**

Cold Sores

SAY THIS

If a canker sore doesn't go away, it could be oral cancer. Catch it early. Check out this save-a-life rap from Eva Grayzel.

"

DESCRIPTION

Eva Grazel tells a great story in a fun way about watching out for canker sores.

LINK: **WWW.RACHELMELE.COM/11-10**

National Pizza Day

SAY THIS

Who here has ever burnt the roof of their mouth on pizza? Ouch that hurts.

#NationalPizzaDay

99

DESCRIPTION

Get pizza for the team! This is another good topic for your blog.

LINK: **WWW.RACHELMELE.COM/11-11**

Child's Teeth

SAY THIS

It's important to care for your child's teeth and (oral) health from birth. Be sure to clean your infant's gums after feedings and don't put your baby to bed with a bottle. Remember dental decay is an infectious transmissible disease. Avoid testing the temperature of the bottle with your mouth, sharing utensils or cleaning a pacifier by putting it in your mouth.

"

DESCRIPTION

This is informational enough to turn it into a quick 30 second video or blog explaining how to take care of baby's teeth.

LINK: **WWW.RACHELMELE.COM/11-12**

National Diabetes Day

SAY THIS

In honor of National Diabetes Day, here's Joey Fatone reminding us about good oral health.

"

DESCRIPTION

Link in your post to this fun Colgate commercial with Joey Fatone giving dental advice.

LINK: WWW.RACHELMELE.COM/11-13

Contest

SAY THIS

*What are you thankful for? Fill out a
leaf at your next appointment and place it
on our tree or post below. You could win
two tickets to the movies.*

"

DESCRIPTION

If you don't want to put up a tree for
the leafs to go in, they could be placed
in a box or hung on the wall, etc.

LINK: **WWW.RACHELMELE.COM/11-14**

Practice Map

Here is a map to our practice to share with your friends. How many different ways can you get to our office?

,,

DESCRIPTION

The link below takes you to instructions for creating a link to your office map.

LINK: **WWW.RACHELMELE.COM/11-15**

Insurance Reminder

SAY THIS

It's almost the end of the year. Don't forget to use your dental benefits before year's end. Our year-end schedule is nearly full, so be sure to call us soon.

[Practice Phone #]

"

DESCRIPTION

Allow for appointment openings for patients that need to use their end of year Health Savings Account and insurance balance.

LINK: WWW.RACHELMELE.COM/11-16

NOVEMBER 17TH

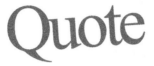

SAY THIS

"A smile will gain you ten more years of life."

~Chinese Proverb @KnightandHammer

DESCRIPTION

Post a smile from ear to ear.

LINK: **WWW.RACHELMELE.COM/11-17**

Dental TV Scene

SAY THIS

Anyone watch Full House? We love this dental scene:

"

DESCRIPTION

Popular movies and TV shows with dental scenes can be a great way to engage patients on social media.

LINK: WWW.RACHELMELE.COM/11-18

Thanksgiving

SAY THIS

Who says it's no fun at the kid's table!? Check out these awesome Thanksgiving snack ideas for kids and adults alike!

,,

DESCRIPTION

Attach a photo and consider adding your own suggestions to your blog.

LINK: WWW.RACHELMELE.COM/11-19

Mannequin Challenge

SAY THIS

We have created a mannequin challenge video. We hope you have as much fun watching it as we had making it.

"

DESCRIPTION

Include as many of the team members as you can in this fun exercise where everyone freezes like they are in a photo but it's all on video.

LINK: WWW.RACHELMELE.COM/11-20

Thanksgiving

SAY THIS

Today everyone is getting ready for their great feast.
Here is some preparation fun.

99

DESCRIPTION

Can you think of a way to
portray this comic in your own
way? How about swapface?

LINK: WWW.RACHELMELE.COM/11-21

Thanksgiving

SAY THIS

[Practice Doctor(s)] Thanksgiving dinner table is all set! Who's hungry?

,,

DESCRIPTION

Post a picture of a dinner place setting with toothbrush, toothpaste, floss, mouth rinse added as utensils.

LINK: **WWW.RACHELMELE.COM/11-22**

We are Thankful for...

SAY THIS

Here at [Practice Name], we are so incredibly thankful for our amazing patients.

"

DESCRIPTION

Create your own image of all the things your practice has to be thankful.

LINK: WWW.RACHELMELE.COM/11-23

Patient Appreciation

SAY THIS

Thank you for being such great patients. To show our appreciation, we invite you and your friends to come to the movies on us. See information below.

,,

DESCRIPTION

Rent out the movie theater for the Saturday after Thanksgiving when all the new movies come out.

LINK: WWW.RACHELMELE.COM/11-24

Continuing Education

SAY THIS

[Practice Name] is dedicated to continuing education. Today, we are attending [Meeting Attending]. We are always looking for ways to make things better for you.

"

DESCRIPTION

Share the enthusiasm of learning together.

LINK: **WWW.RACHELMELE.COM/11-25**

National Flossing Day

SAY THIS

Today is the day you have all been waiting for. No excuses today. It's National Flossing Day! Show us your flossing pics.

"

DESCRIPTION

Take a video or post a picture of everyone in your office flossing.

LINK: WWW.RACHELMELE.COM/11-26

Tooth Fairy

SAY THIS

In France, the "tooth fairy" is a mouse!

"

DESCRIPTION

Ask a patient to draw a picture of a mouse tooth fairy and post it on social media.

LINK: WWW.RACHELMELE.COM/11-27

Specialist Contest

SAY THIS

We challenged our dental specialist offices to create the "best" ornament. Vote for the one you like best, and that office will win lunch on us!

99

DESCRIPTION

This is a fun way to promote your specialists and increase your followers.

LINK: **WWW.RACHELMELE.COM/11-28**

Gum Disease

SAY THIS

Whoopi Goldberg talks about gum disease – It can kill you!

,,

DESCRIPTION

Link to this video of Whoopi on YouTube.

LINK: **WWW.RACHELMELE.COM/11-29**

Dental Fun

SAY THIS

We want to see your before and after Movember shots. What do you think, does [Practice Doctor(s)] look better with or without a mustache?

,,

DESCRIPTION

You can have followers vote on social media. Be sure to respond to every post.

LINK: **WWW.RACHELMELE.COM/11-30**

Patient Recognition

SAY THIS

Here is December's Smile of the Month!

,,

DESCRIPTION

Choose patients that have a great smile and also a talent. Get permission from patient to post.

LINK: WWW.RACHELMELE.COM/12-1

Decorations

SAY THIS

The [Practice Name] office is all decorated for the Holidays. Do you have your decorations up yet? 〞

DESCRIPTION

Followers will enjoy your page more with unique fun posts mixed with informational posts.

LINK: WWW.RACHELMELE.COM/12-2

National Cookie Day

SAY THIS

To celebrate National Cookie Day, all our patients who have appointments or stop by today will get a tooth cookie.

"

DESCRIPTION

Get your cookie cutter online.

LINK: **WWW.RACHELMELE.COM/12-3**

Food Drive

SAY THIS

We are putting together a food/toy drive that will run for a week, ending with a party. There is a raffle for every 5 items donated.

"

DESCRIPTION

Take a photo of your team behind all the food/toys you have collected thus far or a photo from last year.

LINK: **WWW.RACHELMELE.COM/12-4**

Contest

SAY THIS

The [Practice Name] team is having a dental themed Christmas tree contest. You and your friends can vote on your favorite tree, and we'll donate a [Prize] to the winning team member's charity of choice.

99

DESCRIPTION

Use models of teeth, gloves, toothbrushes and more to create different dental themed Christmas trees. Number your trees for easy follower voting.

LINK: WWW.RACHELMELE.COM/12-5

Informational

SAY THIS

What makes something beautiful? This dentist, Jane Weavis, "takes beauty down to the basics" in this video revealing underlying mathematical truths about our smiles.

,,

DESCRIPTION

Encourage your patients to make their smiles more "beautiful."

LINK: **WWW.RACHELMELE.COM/12-6**

Team Appreciation

SAY THIS

We are proud to say that our practice team has over [# of years] of experience.

99

DESCRIPTION

Add all the years of dental experience your team members have.

LINK: WWW.RACHELMELE.COM/12-7

Dental Fun

SAY THIS

*Trying to decide what present to get for your kids for the holidays? How about a Barbie Careers Dentist playset? This was [Practice Doctor(s)] favorite toy growing up. *smile**

,,

DESCRIPTION

Great interested patients make great interested employees when they grow up.

LINK: WWW.RACHELMELE.COM/12-8

Toy Drive

SAY THIS

We are doing a Holiday Toy Drive. Please help us support the Toys for Tots Foundation and bring in an unopened toy.

"

DESCRIPTION

You can make a difference.

LINK: WWW.RACHELMELE.COM/12-9

Stay Healthy

SAY THIS

This is the time of year our diets tend to get out of whack. Here are some tips to help stay healthy.

,,

DESCRIPTION

This is a great blog topic and you could also print and have the information available at the front office.

LINK: WWW.RACHELMELE.COM/12-10

Toothbrush

SAY THIS

What's your preference, manual or electric toothbrush? Which kind do you think [Practice Doctor(s)] uses?

,,

DESCRIPTION

Respond to follower postings in a timely fashion.

LINK: WWW.RACHELMELE.COM/12-11

Ugly Sweater

SAY THIS

[Practice Doctor(s)] got a new sweater. What do you think?

,,

DESCRIPTION

Purchase an ugly dentist themed sweater like this one and post a picture of the doctor wearing it.

LINK: WWW.RACHELMELE.COM/12-12

Dental App

SAY THIS

Clean Santa's teeth with this fun

dental app.

,,

DESCRIPTION

Link straight to the game on iTunes or create a video of [Practice Doctor(s)] playing the app himself.

LINK: **WWW.RACHELMELE.COM/12-13**

Dental Implants

What are the pros and cons of dental implants?

99

DESCRIPTION

Explain and promote services provided by your practice.

LINK: WWW.RACHELMELE.COM/12-14

National Cupcake Day

SAY THIS

In honor of National Cupcake Day, all of today's patients will get a tooth-shape cupcake. Don't have an appointment today? Stop by anyway.

,,

DESCRIPTION

Here are instructions to make tooth shaped cupcakes or if you don't want to make them yourself, ask the local baker.

LINK: WWW.RACHELMELE.COM/12-15

Twitter

SAY THIS

[Practice Name] has a Twitter account. Follow us on [Twitter address].

,,

DESCRIPTION

Include a Twitter Logo in your post.

LINK: WWW.RACHELMELE.COM/12-16

Insurance

SAY THIS

Is there something about your smile you'd like to fix before the insurance year is out? We're here for you, but our schedule is filling up fast! Call us today at [Practice Phone Number] or request your appointment online. Here is a calendar for you to help with your planning.

"

DESCRIPTION

Grab a blank calendar (or print one from online). Write in one of the calendar dates "Make my Smile Great" and then circle it in red.

LINK: **WWW.RACHELMELE.COM/12-17**

Holiday Cards

SAY THIS

Thank you to everyone who has sent us a holiday card! Please keep them coming.

"

DESCRIPTION

Take a photo of all your holiday cards posted on the office wall.

LINK: WWW.RACHELMELE.COM/12-18

Elf on the Shelf

SAY THIS

Look who showed up today in our brushing area.

--- 99 ---

DESCRIPTION

You can have lots of fun with the "elf" on Facebook this month. Be creative.

LINK: WWW.RACHELMELE.COM/12-19

Stocking Stuffers

SAY THIS

What's your favorite dental stocking stuffer? Here are some ideas:

"

DESCRIPTION

Take a picture of a stocking filled with hygiene supplies.

LINK: WWW.RACHELMELE.COM/12-20

Toy Drive

SAY THIS

Look, Santa! [Practice Doctor(s)] and his elves stopped by our office to support our toy drive.

"

DESCRIPTION

Dress up like Santa (or put a Santa hat on) and take a picture with the collected toys.

LINK: WWW.RACHELMELE.COM/12-21

Holiday

SAY THIS

Happy Holidays from
[Practice Name].

99

DESCRIPTION

Upload videos to jibjab.com of each staff member in a Happy Holidays ecard to patients.

LINK: **WWW.RACHELMELE.COM/12-22**

Dental Fun

SAY THIS

*"All I want for Christmas is My Two Front Teeth"
was written by Donald Gardner in 1944. He asked
his second-grade class what they wanted for
Christmas, and noticed that almost all of the
students had at least one front tooth missing as
they answered in a lisp. Gardner wrote the song in
30 minutes. Happy Holidays everyone!*

99

DESCRIPTION

Post the link to Wikipedia, a YouTube video to
a kiddo singing about two front teeth or get
one of your patients without two front teeth
to do a video for you.

LINK: **WWW.RACHELMELE.COM/12-23**

Holiday Party

SAY THIS

*Here's our practice celebrating a great
year with awesome patients at our annual
Holiday party.*

,,

DESCRIPTION

Display a picture of the team dressed up at
your Holiday party, if you have one.

LINK: WWW.RACHELMELE.COM/12-24

Merry Christmas

SAY THIS

Do you know how much sugar your child eats? Check out this article from Parents Magazine and remember today is National Brush Day.

"

DESCRIPTION

Create your own graphic, make it representative of your practice.

LINK: WWW.RACHELMELE.COM/12-25

Practice Promotion

SAY THIS

You are never too old to have a beautiful smile and we can help. Make it a New Year's resolution.

Call our office at [Telephone #].

,,

DESCRIPTION

Feature one of your mature patients who achieved great results.

LINK: WWW.RACHELMELE.COM/12-26

Tooth Fairy

SAY THIS

Have you seen the best Tooth Fairy ever? Check it out.

"

DESCRIPTION

Participate in local fairs and support local organizations.

LINK: WWW.RACHELMELE.COM/12-27

Quote

SAY THIS

"A smile starts on the lips. A grin spreads to the eyes. A chuckle comes from the belly. But a good laugh bursts forth from the soul, overflows and bubbles all around" ~Carolyn Birmingham. Here are some baby laughs from our receptionist, [Practice Team Member]'s little one.

99

DESCRIPTION

Recreate this cute YouTube video
or just link to the original.

LINK: WWW.RACHELMELE.COM/12-28

Dental Fun

SAY THIS

How often do you change your toothbrush? Don't be like this guy.

"

DESCRIPTION

In this Colgate® video, a seriously disgusting toothbrush takes over.

LINK: WWW.RACHELMELE.COM/12-29

Resolutions

SAY THIS

Are you thinking about your New Year's resolutions? Make it a better smile.

,,

DESCRIPTION

Guide your patients to help them make good dental decisions.

LINK: WWW.RACHELMELE.COM/12-30

Happy New Year

SAY THIS

Happy New Year, everyone! What is your resolution for 20[ ]? We wish you a happy, healthy and successful year ahead!

,,

DESCRIPTION

Take a picture of team members and create a collage of friendly faces.

LINK: WWW.RACHELMELE.COM/12-31

Made in the USA
Coppell, TX
07 September 2020

36389857R00207